DIE

Arrest

"The lessons of this compelling and amazing story apply to every community in the United States."

Mickey S. Eisenberg, M.D., Ph. D, author of *Life in the Balance*

"A poignant, touching glimpse of the inner workings of a family impacted by cardiac arrest. This is a must read for heart patients and their loved ones."

Wayne M. Sotile, Ph.D., author of *Thriving with Heart Disease*

"It makes you laugh, it makes you cry; it has everything. The descriptions are so interesting. It is fast paced, the action and details capture you."

Mary Newman, President, Sudden Cardiac Arrest Foundation

A HEART TOO GOOD TO DIE

A shocking story of Sudden Cardiac Arrest

Jeremy Whitehead

Foreword by David A. Rubin M.D.

A HEART TOO GOOD TO DIE is a work of nonfiction.
It is based on the recollections of the author and witnesses.

Printed in the United States of America.

This publication contains the opinions and experiences of the author.
It is intended to provide helpful and informative material on the
subjects addressed in the publication. It is not intended to be a
substitute for professional medical advice, diagnosis, or treatment.
Always seek the advice of your physician or other qualified health
provider with any questions you may have regarding a medical
condition.

The author gratefully acknowledges permission to reprint material:
Dr. Larry Dossey, *Healing Words: The Power of Prayer and the Practice of
Medicine*, HarperCollins, 1993.

Library of Congress Control Number: 2007910291

ISBN 978-1-60145-408-9

Booklocker.com, Inc.
2008

*For Carolyn, she missed so much
and yet she endured it all.*

Contents

FOREWORD

Carolyn Whitehead was one of the few—*is* one of the very few—lucky ones. She not only survived an out-of-hospital cardiac arrest, but regained full use of her faculties. Despite all the improvements in the detection and treatment of heart disease, over 300,000 people have died each year, and will die of sudden death in the next year. Before the advent of bystander CPR and paramedic teams equipped with automatic external defibrillators, the chance of survival was less than 5%. Carolyn had the good fortune to sustain her episode in the presence of two people trained in CPR, and a team equipped with a defibrillator quickly arrived. Even so, her chances of survival without significant brain damage were less than one in four. She had all the predictors of a poor outcome: arrest duration more than 15 minutes, hypotension, tracheal intubation, and coma. Her story is truly remarkable.

Her story is also unusual. Although sudden death is the initial presentation of heart disease in nearly half the patients, there is usually some identifiable underlying disease. In the United States, the most common cause, accounting for roughly 80% of cardiac arrests, is coronary artery disease—thus the initial thoughts of her treating physicians. The second leading cause is thickening of the heart muscle (left ventricular hypertrophy). In the United States, hypertension is the most common cause of left ventricular hypertrophy. There are also rare inheritable disorders of the heart muscle that can cause abnormal thickening of the heart muscle, termed hypertropic cardiomyopathy. The third most common cause is cardiomyopathy, a weakening of the heart muscle that can affect either the squeezing out of the blood to the rest of the body (systolic dysfunction), or the relaxation of the heart muscle that allows the blood to enter the heart (diastolic dysfunction).

Lastly there are disorders of the ion currents that control the electrical activity of the heart. These disorders can lead to short circuits that cause rapid, ineffectual contractions of the heart muscle that result in collapse.

Carolyn had none of the above, as proved by the extensive but ultimately frustrating evaluation by her extremely competent team of physicians. Carolyn is an excellent and unfortunate example of what we do *not* know about disorders of the heart.

She is, however, the beneficiary of therapy that we do know prevents recurrence of cardiac arrest. Unlike lightning, cardiac arrest *will* hit the same place twice. Studies report a recurrence rate of 50-60% at two years. Drugs have been relatively ineffective in the prevention of recurrences. The introduction of implantable defibrillators has revolutionized the care of cardiac arrest survivors. These devices detect the cardiac arrest and automatically deliver a shock to terminate the arrhythmia. The devices are extremely effective, but they are not without their shortcomings. The recalls due to defects in battery and lead design are now, unfortunately, commonplace news headlines. There are risks attendant with the implantation, including collapsed lungs, heart perforations and infections. Fortunately, the recalls and complications are rare.

Carolyn's story also illustrates the non-medical complications of cardiac arrest and its therapy—the social and psychological problems. Cardiac arrest is a life changing experience for both the patient and her family. Mr. Whitehead delineates these problems in a passionate, yet lucid and empathetic manner.

Thus, Carolyn's story, as told by her husband, has a lesson for many people. It is instructive to patients who have survived cardiac arrest and have not come to grips with the emotional trauma. It is instructive to family members and friends who have to deal with a loved one who has survived cardiac arrest. And, yes, her story has something for those of us who deal with sudden death victims. I gained insight into the struggles of families dealing with such a catastrophic event, and how we as physicians appear to families. I have cared for Carolyn for the past few years. Yet, it is only now, through this book, that I believe that I truly know Carolyn and her husband.

Lastly, this story is a lesson in love—the love of a husband for his wife, the love of a brother for his sister, and the love of friends and colleagues for a remarkable person. This is a lesson of value to us all.

David. A. Rubin, M.D.
Clinical Professor of Medicine
Columbia University College of Physicians and Surgeons
November 2007

INTRODUCTION

When sudden cardiac death strikes, there is nothing you can do. Nothing the spouse can do, nothing the family can do, and nothing best friends or colleagues at work can do. It just takes them away, around nine out of ten victims, and it takes them in minutes. They do not come back. They are gone. But it doesn't have to be that way. They can survive, and become "hearts too good to die".

Most die before reaching the hospital, and it happens to outwardly healthy people with no known heart problems such as high school kids, college sports stars and professional athletes, as well as thousands of children.

Sometimes there is a warning sign, but often there is not. You would be surprised if your favorite nightly news station reported the cases—over ten times more deaths than car fatalities—nearly one thousand per day in the United States alone. When this "serial killer" strikes, it is usually not gruesome, and yet it is sudden and shocking, so why don't we hear about these tragedies?

Even if we did hear about them more, what could you do? How do you deal with a sudden cardiac arrest? Cardiopulmonary resuscitation will not bring them back, although it may keep them going long enough for the one thing that will save them.

They need a defibrillator.

To shock them back to life.

Dick Cheney has one; his cardiologist thinks he is in danger without one. Reggie Lewis and Hank Gathers didn't know they needed one. An external one could have saved Sergei Grinkov on the ice rink.

Those that survive are changed forever. Most likely an expensive device, similar to a pacemaker, will be implanted in their chest. The spouses, family and friends will all be impacted. Who helps them? Where do they get the information and support to deal with the changes? The facts are easy to come by, often too plentiful, and yet so uninformative. There are few books that tell the story, or offer to educate and explain without a clinical approach.

We want to understand what is happening, what will happen next, and how to prepare for the future.

༄

For the survivors and family, emotions run high. Grief is not far away and yet we need to be prepared for the implant procedure to be performed "in a few days time", and the subsequent invasive tests. Too often, the advice is preoccupied with prevention, rather than the rehabilitation and recuperation we all need—for the mind as much as the body. Even though the emotions are often buried, they resurface and the questions start all over again. Why did this happen? What does it mean? Will they recover? How do we deal with it?

I had very little information, with even less experience, and even today, it still feels unreal.

Carolyn had arrhythmias for over twenty years; mild and annoying irregularities in her heartbeat, sometimes as a result of strenuous exercise or periods of high emotion. The technical term is Premature Ventricular Contractions (but always called PVCs) and to her it felt like "a pause, then thump" at the wrong time. No big deal, sometimes she put up with hundreds of them in a day, and never did they interfere with her quality of life.

That was not the case in October 2002. With odds of ten million to one, a PVC landing at just the wrong time would do it. *It* happened while she was sitting down, having just introduced herself to a large group of co-workers at a management seminar. She fainted and fell out of her chair—a big surprise to those around her.

She had suffered a sudden cardiac arrest. Her heart was not pumping blood, she was not breathing, and her brain was not getting any oxygen. She was clinically dead.

Introduction

This book can help those of you who have faced the trauma of sudden cardiac arrest in your circle. I sought just such a book when confronting my wife's medical emergency, but could find few similar stories, and they did not address the topic of sudden cardiac arrest directly.

Candidates for an Implantable Cardioverter Defibrillator, and their families, have many unanswered questions. I still face despair and confusion over what happened to my wife that October morning. Maybe it will never go away. Knowing more helps, but sharing the feelings and experience has certainly aided the healing.

This is a story of a medical emergency, seen from the eyes of a spouse. Close friends and colleagues should find familiarity and comfort in these words too. The practitioners do not always handle us very well, even when our services are required. I do not lay any blame; they too are not necessarily well informed. Their job is to diagnose and remedy the physical damage presented—the pathology. Medicine is a science, and has rules to operate by. Our job is to support and nurture our loved ones' will to survive; without it, they don't stand a chance. You and your survivor will find much joy and fulfillment in your "new" relationship, with extraordinarily tender moments and intense closeness, purely because they are still here, against the odds.

Chapter 1

IN GOOD COMPANY

Great crises produce great men, and great deeds of courage.
—John F. Kennedy

It was the most frightening time of my life. Nothing had prepared me for the responsibility or the dread. That precious heart had to be stilled. An electric shock would do the job. Only a small shock, but delivered at just the right time and in exactly the right place. She would be dead; there would be no pulse, and thus no life giving oxygen for her brain and organs. Her blood pressure and heart rhythm had to be monitored to ensure the precise conditions were achieved. But first she must be sedated so she would not feel any pain, or suffer in any way.

Naturally, I was apprehensive and worried. Their reasoning was unequivocal. It was vitally important—her life depended on it!

How could this be possible? What justification could there be for terminating my beautiful wife's heartbeat? She was young, fit and healthy—normal in every respect. Why should she succumb to this hideous proposition? And how could a spouse be asked to sanction such a grave act?

To find out we should start at the beginning; to the first time she dies.

Carolyn and I were newly married and had left Australia to begin a wonderful new life together in America. We had grand plans, and I felt lucky to be accepted into this land of opportunity. Our home was now Boston, Massachusetts, and I was still adjusting to my new surroundings when Carolyn had to leave for Texas. She had no indication that this routine business trip would have such a dire outcome. Neither did I, so the phone call from Dallas was both alarming and confusing—it left me terrified.

I had expected our wedding day to be the highlight of my New England experience. Thursday, October 10th, 2002 has now been permanently imprinted in my mind. It was mid morning when the call came on the home phone—the one the telemarketers had already found. It wouldn't have been Carolyn, as she preferred to ring my cell phone, which had all those free minutes we paid for every month! The caller was no stranger, although we had never spoken before. Unquestionably, he had shocking news.

"Is that Jeremy Whitehead?"

"Yes, speaking." A chill passed down my spine. Nobody ever starts a telephone call that way unless....

"This is Jim Hardee, Carolyn's boss. Your wife's had a bit of a turn, and we've taken her to the hospital. I think you should get down here."

"Get down where?" I wondered, although I should have known. Carolyn had left the previous day for the conference in Dallas and we had spoken just a few hours earlier to say good morning; a small ritual of love we used to help bridge the physical distance.

Jim had been Carolyn's boss just a few months. He had taken a bold step in hiring her as a Business Unit Executive, just before the summer. We were both in the IT industry, successfully climbing the corporate ladder in Australia. I was in sales and marketing, and she was a regional manager. But Carolyn had found an opportunity to advance to "the next level", leading a sales team with revenue targets in the hundreds of millions of dollars. She matched the job requirements perfectly, although there had been an underlying sentiment of, "how could someone all the way from Australia be successful in this role?" Unperturbed, Carolyn had proven herself within a few short weeks to be an inspirational leader, motivating her team to overachieve, as well as boosting morale to an all time high. But now, Jim was calling to say there was some problem with her health, and he seemed worried.

Maybe Carolyn had overreacted to a minor ailment like an upset stomach, cramp or a bad headache. I was always teasing her about her low tolerance to physical pain, so I was embarrassed to hear Jim say they had sent her to the hospital. He and I had not met, but Carolyn had talked about him enough for me to feel that I knew him. Alas, he did not feel the same way.

"Oh I don't think that will be necessary," I blurted out, while trying to work out where on earth Dallas was. I knew it was in Texas, but how far is that from Boston? Do I drive? Maybe a plane is better. Oh, how will I get a ticket? Who do I call? I was very used to sudden travel demands back home. The Qantas Club membership had made those types of dramas so easy to handle. Alone, in our rental apartment in Boston, I had my morning planned out and was busy getting my tasks done. Until that moment.

"Maybe you should talk to the doctor," Jim replied.

I felt a bag of icy water land in the pit of my stomach. Doctor? What doctor?

"This is Dr. Diamond from Baylor Grapevine emergency ward, your wife has been admitted to intensive care in critical condition." He paused, letting those words sink in before continuing, "We are not sure what happened to her, but she has had a cardiac arrest, maybe due to an aneurism. She is stable right now, and we should know more in twelve hours or so."

My legs were suddenly weak; they buckled. The bag of icy water had broken and, now sitting on the floor, I wondered what could have happened to my bride.

Did he really say those terrifying words "critical condition"?

I wanted to be sick, I wasn't breathing, and my stomach somehow knew what my brain was attempting to deny.

❧

Carolyn and the three managers who reported to her, Pam Battistone, Bruce Senecal and Karen Davey, were part of a group of over two hundred attending a high performance management conference, as part of

their IBM leadership development program. Carolyn had little chance
to notice how well the Hilton Dallas Fort Worth Lakes Executive Conference Center specialized in such conferences. That morning they had
numerous rooms allocated to handle the large influx of IBMers. The
rooms were configured to accommodate groups of thirty people, each
with four tables set for the morning's activity. A table captain had been
assigned in advance; a little surprise for four of the best. This was going
to be their office for the next two days.

Karen did not think there was anything amiss with Carolyn that
Thursday morning. The four of them had met in the lobby to go down
for breakfast together. "When we travel, we travel in packs" was her
maxim. Carolyn seemed quiet, but they hadn't spent much time that
early in the morning before, and Karen was still getting to know her
new leader, so she accepted that Carolyn was not her usual self.

They found their way down to the auditorium; the basement level
of the hotel was like a maze but the corridors were full of people
headed for the same location. Karen had learned that her boss liked to
sit up front and on the aisle, so they filed into one of the front rows.
After hearing about the day's agenda, they were organized into groups
and dispersed to the conference rooms. Another flight of stairs and
winding passages brought them into a room with round tables; eight
places each set with nametags, pitchers of water and bowls of candy.

Karen noticed that Carolyn had been pre-selected as table captain,
and that Bruce was assigned the seat next to her. Karen was bound for
a different table, however, and was thus among strangers. Everything
went according to plan, until they were in the middle of the normal
"show and tell" get-to-know-you session. Karen's table had been first to
do the introductions, and she was watching Bruce as he stood up to
begin his story.

Bruce felt well rested, as they had had an early evening the night
before. The previous day had been long, the flight in from Boston providing an extra hour with the change in time zone, but having dinner
with the three girls was fun; they had had a few drinks, and lots of

laughs. He liked this opportunity to be with them outside the office. But he was surprised to see Carolyn so quiet at breakfast. Nevertheless, they stuck together through the opening session, "as the team we are" he thought to himself. Then the huge group was split into teams for the real business to begin.

It was Tom O'Brien's first time as co-facilitator and, wanting to make a stimulating and fresh start, he decided to add a twist to the standard course opening. Hoping to make the introductions interesting, he asked each person to describe something no one else would know about them.

Tom was pleased with the early results, as the attendees were a little challenged by the request and thus paying attention. It was going to be a memorable session.

As a Certified Professional Coach and Sales Transformation Manager, and based in Fort Worth, Texas, Sara Smith was technically in charge of the training session. She enjoyed having the chance to watch the group from the back of the room; normally she was out front doing the talking, but this time she could listen and observe. She felt comfortable with Tom leading, although neither of them realized how they would be tested by the forthcoming events.

Bruce was not especially thrilled to have to stand up and reveal something about himself to these "strangers". And having to wait for his turn was an unbearable torture. With eight per table there was plenty of time for the stress to build up, and he couldn't stop the mantra in his head, "What is it that I'm going to say?"

Each time someone got up and told their story he changed his mind, and had to search for something new. Karen had surprised everyone with her story about being expert at throwing the javelin. How could he beat that? There was one thing he could reveal, but that would probably be too revealing. He was sitting next to Carolyn, and realized that he had better decide quickly. Once she was finished with her introduction it would be his turn.

Jim knew them all, and being a Vice President he had been able to arrange for his entire management team to be in the one room. Introductions were a normal part of these types of business meetings; he was listening, but not really paying attention. He had other things on his mind, thinking about how this course would help his team to uncover and resolve problems on the front lines.

Mark Johnson was sitting in the back of the room observing the introductions. It was rare to have all of the team in one place and he saw this as an opportunity to build rapport with them. He saw Carolyn stand up to speak and was enthralled in her unique story. As the Human Resources manager for Jim's team, Mark had been involved in Carolyn's recruitment. She was no stranger, but not yet well known to him. That was about to change forever.

Randy Fitch was sitting seven or eight feet away from Carolyn; her table was in front of his and over to one side. As each group introduced themselves, Randy moved his chair to face their table. He was particularly interested to learn that Carolyn was able to communicate via sign language, and yet she was not deaf and neither were any of her family. She stood up straight and moved her hands and fingers as she spoke, demonstrating her skill. It was a surprising trait and certainly memorable. The girls seemed to have the edge with the revelations, first a javelin thrower and then a hearing person that signs. As Jim's executive assistant, Randy had both an envious and challenging role. He's a cool-customer, very direct and forthright; not so much a hard taskmaster, but determined and disciplined—a man of actions rather than words.

Watching Carolyn as she sat down, Randy was glad his table already had their turn. Surprisingly, he was feeling a little clammy. "Probably just nerves. There is an element of risk here. This is an embarrassing thing to do," he told himself, and then sought to rationalize it: "Having to stand up and speak to a large group of people and reveal something new about yourself can be stressful." He could not have predicted just how stressful that morning was going to be.

Bruce had just stood up and opened his mouth to speak, when Carolyn collapsed at his feet. She just slid off her chair and fell to the floor like a bag of potatoes, not quite graceful, almost gentle; a crumpling as opposed to a thud.

Randy sensed it happening in slow motion and thought, "I should be trying to catch her." He knew she was going down—somehow before she fell—possibly from instinct. Time had slowed down, but his mind was running at a million miles per hour. He was not quick enough, however, and she was already on the floor before he was even out of his chair.

Standing at the front of the room, Tom could easily see everyone and was surprised when Carolyn slid off her chair. "She couldn't have fallen asleep," he thought, "maybe she slipped."

Jim was shocked to see her fall, and thought, "Oh, I hope she's just fainted." Not sure what was going on, he wanted to know if it was serious or not. "I can't believe it is anything more than that, I have to go to her."

But it was much more than that.

Although Sara was at the back of the room, she had a clear view of Carolyn. She saw the energy drain out of Carolyn's body, leaving a face devoid of expression—just blank. All of Carolyn's muscles suddenly went slack, like cutting the strings to a puppet, and she dropped to the floor.

Randy's first thought was that Carolyn had fainted, maybe due to a chemical imbalance in her blood; being hypoglycemic, Randy knew the feeling. Once before, he had been in a meeting where someone had fainted, but this time he was uncertain, for there had been no warning, no gasps or moans, just silence until the thump.

Sitting at the adjacent table, Karen also guessed that Carolyn had fainted and feared that she may have hurt herself in the fall, as she herself had experienced a few years back. Even though Carolyn had been sitting down, she could have hit her head or banged her nose. Knowing that she was not going to be of any use medically, Karen rushed outside to alert someone. Looking back into the room she saw several people were already attending to Carolyn on the floor. She decided to approach everyone she met on her way to find the conference command center, and ask whether they had any medical training.

When Carolyn hit the floor, Mark stood up. He could see Tom and Randy rush over to her. All the panicked faces at the front of the room told him something serious had occurred, and his first instinct was to get help. He raced over to the back door of the room, and out into the corridor.

Randy reached Carolyn first; she was curled up in a fetal position facing away from him. He put his hand on her shoulder, called out her name and then rolled her over. She looked asleep or heavily intoxicated, but there was something else, something not quite right. He could see she was "not there"—completely lifeless and not breathing.

"She's having some kind of episode, and is not waking up," he said to himself as much as to anyone else. Having spent a number of years as a policeman in a county North West of Atlanta, Randy had some experience with emergency situations. He remembered all those car accidents, heart attacks, and stabbings from long ago.

"Carolyn, wake up!" Randy bellowed. His training had kicked in instinctively, and he remembered that yelling into a victim's face was the best way to clearly establish consciousness. As he shouted, he carefully watched her face, hoping to spot just a fluttering of her eyes, or a flinch. There was no response, no reaction. There was no life.

Tom had trained as a medic in the Army Reserves, and although he had not seen any action in Vietnam, he had felt prepared for it. He did not, however, feel prepared for this encounter. Tom saw Carolyn's face turn blue, and realized this was an emergency. "She's not getting any air," he exclaimed.

Putting his ear to Carolyn's chest, Randy could hear strange, unnatural sounds that were neither breaths, nor a proper heartbeat. But he could hear something, so he tried shaking her and calling her name again. It had no effect.

Less than a minute had passed by the time Jim reached her. He was alarmed by Carolyn's unresponsiveness and the color of her skin. He desperately wanted to see some sign of life. He looked towards Tom, hoping he knew what to do.

Whether it was the right thing or the wrong thing to do, Tom knew they had to do something. It would be better than doing nothing; she could die.

"I can hear something but it doesn't sound right," Randy cried out.

Carolyn then gasped a strangled breath and went limp.

Jim knelt down and held her head and, not knowing what else to do, he mimicked Randy's approach, "Carolyn are you there. Wake up, Carolyn!" His shouts achieved nothing. "I must be able to do something more than this!" he thought. "Okay, I'm not a trained professional in medical matters, but what can I do?" The Boy Scout in him reacted; he put his hand under her neck and tilted her head back, recalling that this would prevent Carolyn from swallowing her tongue. Then the realization hit him, "That's all I know to do."

Randy and Tom couldn't determine what was wrong with Carolyn, as there had been no warning, and nothing obviously untoward, apart from her sudden collapse. Had she had a seizure? Was she epileptic? None of them knew anything about her medical history; most had only just met her that day.

Jim could feel the panic taking over, and searched his mind for an antidote. "What should we do now? What does she need?" he asked himself.

Several people had gotten out of their chairs and moved towards the scene, drawn inexorably closer like iron filings to a magnet. Bruce was still standing at his chair, stunned at the suddenness of Carolyn's fall, and startled by her convulsion at his feet. "Oh my God what is happening to her? What can we do to help?" He remembered seeing her take a candy from the bowl on the table, and called out, "I think she might be choking! I saw her take a candy!" He moved back to let the others get closer as he had never been in an emergency before. Bruce felt useless; a room full of high performance managers, and he had no clue what to do.

Tom immediately checked Carolyn's mouth for obstructions, and found that it was clear, so he tilted her head back a little further, pinched her nose closed and put two big breaths into her mouth. There was a lot of resistance to his breath, "just like the first few puffs when blowing up a balloon," he thought. "Got to get the air in, and get the air out," he recalled from that training in the Army so long ago. He felt for Carolyn's sternum, and pushed down firmly on her ribs several times.

Once before, Tom had performed cardiopulmonary resuscitation in an emergency, (although he had learned to say CPR), and he was willing to do it again. It had been the mid 1980s, also at a training conference, when a colleague had collapsed on the volleyball court. All the IBM managers at that time undertook CPR training, so he was called to assist until the first responders could get there. Unfortunately, it had taken him several minutes to get courtside and his efforts were unsuccessful.

Unsure exactly how many times to pump and how many breaths to blow into her mouth, Tom was more worried about the likelihood that it was not going to do Carolyn any good. He thought his actions might make things worse than they already were; after all, that training so long ago had been perfunctory.

Bruce couldn't stand still any longer; he had do something more to help. "But what?" he wondered. He thought Carolyn may have been on some medication and seeing a purse on the floor he picked it up to check the contents. There were no pills or prescriptions that could give them a clue. He wasn't even sure it was her pocketbook! When he looked down at Carolyn again he couldn't stop the frightening thoughts, "Oh my god I'm witnessing her death! This just isn't fair. Someone like her, she was making such a difference."

Bruce couldn't have this happen right before his eyes, and believing that no one in the room had any medical background, he decided to go and get expert help. He, too, ran out into the hall, and rushed down the corridor. He frantically opened all the doors to the other rooms, hoping to find someone who knew what to do.

"Oh my, her heart must've stopped," Sara whispered to herself. She could hardly speak, having seen the pallor of Carolyn's face and the way she had dropped like a rag doll. Sara had seen the events unfold in slow motion, and yet she was reassured by the speed of Randy's response.

"He's responding in ways that his hands know what he's doing," she muttered. Sara had also been trained in CPR, but seeing how quickly Randy and Tom were tending to Carolyn, she sensed she was not needed. Momentarily stunned by the sudden calamity, Sara was astonished to remember a workshop she and Randy had held in Atlanta, on September 11th, 2001. She realized that all eight participants from that day were together again at this conference!

Recognizing the seriousness of Carolyn's collapse, Sara seized the conference room phone at the back of the room, and immediately called the coordination point for their conference.

"We have a medical emergency! It is a life or death situation, and we need someone who knows CPR now!"

She turned back to the room and saw that Tom and Randy were busy taking care of Carolyn, but everyone else had a "deer in the headlights" look about them. She stepped forward and suggested everyone help move the tables back. She knew they needed something to do; actions to break the mental paralysis, to help them move through the phases of shock.

Seeing Tom begin the CPR, Randy asked if he could help out. He was willing and able to assist, and he knew they had to get Carolyn breathing again.

Tom suggested that Randy do the chest compressions while he continued with the breaths. He presumed someone had called for help; feeling confident that, just as he was playing his part, others would be doing theirs.

Another minute had slipped by with no discernable effect. Jim was still holding Carolyn's head and staring into her eyes, almost pleading for her to wake up. He saw that her eyes remained glassy and vacant. As Randy and Tom continued the compressions and rescue breathing, Jim noticed that Carolyn's chest only moved up and down when Tom breathed into her.

Jim's thoughts collided as he watched in horror, his world closed in and he couldn't hear the noises around him. He couldn't stop the feeling of helplessness. "This is really bad, she is not breathing by herself," Jim thought as he looked up at Tom, and then down into Carolyn's eyes again. "She's leaving us. This can't happen. This is really serious. She's dying."

Jim did not want to acknowledge these thoughts; they had no place in his experience. This youthful executive, with a vibrant personality that belies his many years in that Fortune 100 company, is smart and very deliberate in actions and words. He is a true southern gentleman, with clear blue eyes and a muscular physique that perfectly matches his zeal for sporting activities. Usually very capable and determined, Jim was not used to feeling powerless. But he just didn't know what else they could do.

❦

All was calm outside the conference room, and only a few minutes had passed in what felt like an eternity, when Mark found some hotel office staff down one of the many corridors. He called out, "A person has collapsed in the conference room! We need help!"

Hotel security was alerted, and a middle aged, heavy-set guard came pounding down the corridor, with keys jangling, and walkie-talkie squawking. Mark led the way, and a moment later they were standing at the open door to the room. They saw Carolyn motionless on the floor, surrounded by a crowd of her colleagues watching with a hushed nervousness. A sense of helplessness filled the air.

Moving just a little inside the doorway, Mark could see that Jim was holding Carolyn's head, and that Randy was pushing on her chest, while Tom checked her pulse. One of them said, "She still isn't breathing." Mark tried to blink the image away, but it was so very real. On the next blink he saw Tom blow into her mouth.

"Call 9-1-1, we need an ambulance now," the anxious guard barked into his shoulder microphone.

In another hallway, somebody heard Karen's cry for help, "Do you know where I can find medical help? There's a woman in our room who fell and I think she's passed out!"

The passerby smiled and said, "There's a room full of nurses right around the corner." A nurse's training conference was underway right there in the hotel!

Karen ran down the hall, turned the corner and tried every door she came to.

"Where's the room full of nurses?" she cried.

It was such a maze, and she was anxious that she wouldn't find them in time. She suddenly arrived at the hotel security desk, only to find they already knew about the emergency and had called 9-1-1.

Her single task was now defunct, so Karen ran back towards the room to check on Carolyn's plight. A crowd had formed in the hallway, and she caught snippets of their comments.

"She's not breathing."

"Could be a seizure."

"They're doing CPR on her."

Karen didn't like the sound of this at all. It scared her and she didn't want to see or hear any more. Instead, she found an empty room to escape the tragedy; she was so distraught and just wanted to be alone for a while, to calm down.

❧

Pam's thoughts denied what her eyes revealed. "This is not real, how can it be Carolyn? Why is she the one? She has had such an impact on us, especially me. She has taught us so much." Her clear blue eyes filled with tears as she watched Randy and Tom desperately perform mouth-to-mouth and the chest compressions. Pam was one of the three managers who reported directly to Carolyn, and had spent many hours with her learning how to implement change in the organization, and motivate her team for results. They had been making great progress—until now.

In the past, Pam had witnessed her fair share of drama, but that was to be expected in her previous career—unlike her current job. For several years, she had worked for a national TV news station and vividly remembers the sensationalism and eagerness for action that had overpowered her humanity. She doesn't like to recall that time in the control booth when they cheered as they watched the footage of flames leaping up and consuming someone's house. They had all known the video clip would be highlighted in that evening's news, and had been excited at the prospect.

This time, no one was cheering. This time, she couldn't handle the drama. This was not exhilarating; it was shocking and sudden. It was terrifying to see how quickly and easily life could be extinguished.

Pam recognized that Carolyn was in great danger—people were talking about seizure, epilepsy, her face was blue, and she was making hideous gurgling noises. They were trying to breathe into her mouth, and pushing down hard on her chest.

"This is not fair. We have just got this wonderful person, and she was making a real difference." Pam knew these were selfish thoughts, and felt a little guilty, but they were her real feelings. They could not be ignored.

"Carolyn had so much to give, and was showing us the way forward," Pam thought. She was not ready to say goodbye. Not now, and not like this.

&

While Tom's body was busy blowing into Carolyn's mouth, his mind was considering the three possible outcomes: death, life and the worst possible—living death. "How long has it been?" he wondered. He knew that irreparable damage was likely if the brain was starved of oxygen for more than a few minutes. He also suspected that CPR was not as effective as a real heartbeat in maintaining blood pressure and that critical blood oxygen level.

"How long are we going to continue this? Will *I* have to make the call?" Tom thought. He desperately wanted someone else to tell him when it was the right time to stop. He didn't want that third option to be an option. In the meantime, he continued to breathe for her, as Randy rhythmically thrust down upon her ribcage.

Tom had known someone who remained in a vegetative state for eleven years after surviving a burst blood vessel in her brain. She did not speak, did not see, and did not hear; too many brain cells had been destroyed by the loss of blood flow and the pressure inside her skull. He did not think that survivor had enjoyed "quality of life". He certainly didn't wish that for Carolyn.

What felt like hours had passed in just minutes, and Tom was starting to feel lightheaded. "I'm probably hyperventilating from the constant blowing," he thought. He could see Carolyn's chest rising and falling with each breath, and knew that that was a good sign. If only he could keep going—physically and mentally.

By now, Randy had pushed down on Carolyn's chest several hundred times and, while not quite the same as doing push-ups, he was working up a sweat. He also saw that Tom was finding it hard to get his breath as well as put air into Carolyn's lungs. "Something good should be happening by now, and it isn't," Randy thought, silently and secretly.

9-1-1 had been called. Was there anything more they could do?

❧

Kathy Williams, the passerby to whom Karen had spoken in the hallway, was a little lost in the labyrinth of corridors and rooms. Finding her way back to the nurses' conference, she saw a large group of people standing in the corridor, and instinctively knew they needed help. She wasn't sure if Karen had found anyone to assist, and decided to check.

"What's going on?" she asked.

"Somebody fell down."

"Well, I'm a nurse, let me take a look," Kathy responded.

Entering the room she saw two guys doing a good job of CPR,

although she worried that they might stop. Kathy also heard agonal breathing, and she knew that untrained people could find it hard to pick up on the fact that it was not breathing at all. It was a sign of death in progress, usually a result of the carbon dioxide in the blood reaching a level where the brainstem triggers spontaneous breaths in an effort to re-oxygenate the body.

Tom sensed Kathy standing over him, making an assessment of the situation. She quietly explained that she was a nurse, and offered to help. Tom readily acquiesced.

"Thank God. Now I won't have to make that horrid decision of when to stop," he did not say aloud.

Sara imagined that an angel had just appeared; but it was Kathy that she saw walk into the room and assess the scene in one glance. She heard Kathy say, "Okay, we need to slow down the breaths and increase those beats."

Kathy was clearly worried about their CPR technique, and knelt down beside Tom to take Carolyn's pulse.

"She is exactly what we need right now," Sara thought as she watched Kathy take charge.

"There's some kind of strange flutter going on in her heart," Kathy commented, "and I don't think she is pulling in any air, those gasps are just an automated response." Tom and Randy had paused while Kathy checked for a pulse. While pleased that they had a nurse helping them, they were alarmed that Carolyn was not responding in any way to the CPR.

"She's not breathing on her own," Randy cried out.

He remembered the last time he had to perform CPR in an emergency. It was 1984 and the scene was disturbingly similar to this one. A conference attendee had had a heart attack, and was unconscious on the floor. Randy's first job with IBM was as a security guard, and for thirty minutes he and a registered nurse had worked on this fellow, but they could not save him.

"Oh, no please don't let this happen again," Randy thought. He was unable to stop the feeling of déjà vu. It would not have been helpful for him to know that Tom was thinking the same thing. Neither knew that the other had been unsuccessful with a previous resuscitation effort. It was not something either of them was proud of.

Kathy had much experience with CPR, especially the precariousness of life, and she knew how important it was to be diligent in their efforts. She took over the compressions, counting out the beat so that all three of them would be coordinated. She also made sure that Randy was keeping a careful watch on Carolyn's carotid pulse, to ensure that the compressions were adequate. She wanted to yell out her thoughts, "Someone should go find my friends, I'm in here with a bunch of lay people, and there's a room full of hospital people around here somewhere!" But she did not think that comment would help.

So they continued the CPR, with five breaths to fifteen compressions, four times a minute. It was the correct technique and deemed best for simulating a normal heartbeat and respirations. It was hard work, but having three of them made it less burdensome. On your own it can be frantic and overwhelming, moving from compressions to breaths and most importantly checking for a pulse. It is paramount to stop the cardiac massage if, by miracle, the patient's heart resumes beating. But, there is little likelihood of continuing artificial respiration on a patient that recommences breathing.

Kathy stopped so they could again check for a pulse. There was none, and the color of Carolyn's cheeks hadn't changed from the sickly bluish purple that Tom had first noticed so many minutes earlier.

"Not a healthy color for anyone to be, but with room air it's probably to be expected," Kathy reassured herself. In the hospital she used one hundred percent oxygen which made the patients "pink up nicely."

Randy was relieved that Kathy had taken over the compressions, as her training and experience were greater than his or Tom's; besides they were anxious and tired. They were at their limit and needed the help. If only Carolyn would respond!

More importantly, Kathy knew not to stop before the EMTs

arrived. She knew the occasional gasps and shudders in Carolyn's chest were ineffective. To her, they sounded like a death rattle. She also suspected that Tom and Randy might have stopped if she wasn't there, and then Carolyn would certainly die.

So the resuscitation continued, with Randy checking Carolyn's pulse, Tom carrying on with the breaths and Kathy doing the compressions. They paused every minute or so to see if Carolyn would recover. But when they stopped, the pulse and the breaths stopped too.

Mark was surprised to have seen Kathy stride over and coach Randy and Tom on the correct technique for CPR. He thought it was a lucky coincidence, and felt there could be reason for hope when he saw Kathy encourage them to keep going. He did not know that her thoughts were more extreme.

"We need a defibrillator. For someone this age it has to be a ventricular problem," Kathy thought but did not declare. She didn't know if the hotel had such a device, and although they were standard items in her hospital, not all institutions had yet realized the life saving potential of having them in public places.

She was not the only one in the room who was worried. They had been doing CPR for over ten minutes, and there was no word about the arrival of an ambulance. It was obvious, even to the untrained, that this was too long a time.

With no sign of the emergency services and Carolyn's color stubbornly remaining blue, people started leaving the room in distress, several were trembling and visibly upset.

Mark noticed that hardly anybody was talking, and that several were crying.

"Where are they? I can't hear any sirens, this is taking too long!" Mark silently pleaded. He could not admit the awful realization, "She's dying right here in front of us!"

Seeing the anguish ripple through the group, Sara asked everyone to come out into the hall for a moment. She used some soothing words and once she had their attention she said, "Go outside if you want—

but stay close. When we need to get together again, I'll find you."

Someone asked, "What do we do, now?"

Another replied, "We pray."

And so they waited and prayed. Sara stayed with them to console those who didn't want to be alone. Their grief was apparent, as they each dealt with the tragedy in their own way. Sara was struck by the vision of one manager, a Native American, calling on the spirits to support Carolyn, and realized this was a powerful image for all of them. They needed every form of reassurance, and this indigenous tradition was so special that it could give them all hope.

With everyone ushered out, the doors were closed, but sinister groaning noises escaped from under the door. The minutes now passed so slowly, it seemed like hours.

The prayers were repeated, and more people left the corridor to go outside, unable to accept the dire circumstances they had had to confront so suddenly. What could they do? What will happen to Carolyn? How could this have occurred? *What* had occurred? Their questions remained unanswered.

"Where are they? What is taking them so long? What else can we do?" Bruce questioned himself. He wasn't sure how long the CPR had actually been underway, but it was certainly too long for Carolyn not to be breathing. He did not want to contemplate the consequences. Time was running out, and he felt that her chances were fading with every minute.

∾

Eventually, a faint siren was heard. The Hilton security staff mobilized and cleared a path from the rear of the hotel to the conference center, avoiding the stairways and elevators, thus saving valuable seconds.

Behind the closed door of her private sanctuary, Karen heard the EMTs thunder down the hall. "Oh good, she's going to be all right now," Karen thought, trying to convince herself that they weren't too late. She opened the door and stepped out into the corridor. She was now ready to join the others.

The Grapevine fire rescue paramedics strode past her, pushing a gurney in front of them, with what looked like large plastic toolboxes piled on top. Could they save Carolyn? Had they arrived in time?

∿

The EMS unit that responded to the hotel's emergency 9-1-1 call was Medic 565, a Mobile Intensive Care Unit. These special ambulances are generally dispatched on emergency calls for potentially life threatening episodes, such as unconscious patients, patients with chest pain or those having trouble breathing.

The paramedic on board was trained in Advanced Cardiac Life Support. This qualification includes advanced airway management, the administration of intravenous medications, cardiac monitoring, and defibrillation. The other crewmembers were EMTs, with basic life support training for patient assessment, CPR, bandaging, splinting broken bones, and the administration of oxygen. Together, they operate as a team to perform nearly as effectively as a hospital emergency room. Carolyn was in need of expert emergency care, and these first responders were equipped to handle the situation.

∿

Tom was nearing the limit of his endurance, when suddenly the room filled with uniformed people. The EMTs had surrounded him, with several of the hotel security staff right behind them.

"At last they're here," Tom thought, as he looked up to see the three young men in uniform, one paramedic and two EMTs. He expected them to immediately take over the CPR.

"Oh, that's great. Keep doing that," they told him instead.

When Paramedic Jeff Jackson and EMT Chris Lammons first entered the room, they suspected the worst. Chris had seen many victims in situations like this and, despite all their training and equipment, had had limited success. Their preliminary assessment confirmed that Carolyn was clinically dead. She had all the hallmarks of death——loss of consciousness, no pulse, no blood pressure, and no reaction to stimuli. Although they saw her chest rising and falling, it was obvious she was not breathing on her own. It was only the CPR that was keeping her organs alive. Even to the trained eye, she appeared dead, with only a fleeting chance for survival; biological death would occur within minutes if they couldn't restart her heart. They knew they had to start bagging her; using a handheld squeeze bag to force air into her lungs was better than mouth to mouth, although it would not be enough to revive her.

Chris, the EMT, asked Kathy to describe what had transpired, while Jeff began unpacking their equipment. He was listening intently to her answer as Jeff put the items on the floor next to Carolyn; a BVM airway bag, a silver and green striped oxygen bottle, a long plastic tube in a cellophane wrapper and some syringes. Moving around Tom to do a more thorough inspection, Chris noted the time and that Carolyn was unresponsive with no visible trauma. Her ear, nose and throat were clear, but she had no pulse, no respirations, fixed and dilated pupils, and her skin was cyanotic. Only then did Chris take over the CPR from Tom, placing the BVM mask over Carolyn's mouth and squeezing the reservoir bag quite quickly with his hand.

All signs up to that point indicated sudden cardiac arrest, of unknown cause, and the paramedic expected the cardiac monitor would confirm his suspicions. He noticed how young and slim the patient looked; he didn't know her age but her skin was clear and fresh. She did not seem to be a typical cardiac patient. Despite her apparent health, he could see that the CPR was not going to "bring her back".

There are several forms of pulse-less electrical activity; the most common is ventricular fibrillation, usually abbreviated to "V-fib", or just "VF". There is only one way to stop this deadly arrhythmia—it is not CPR, or drugs—only the life saving shock from a defibrillator. Kathy had known that, and she was relieved to see that the EMTs had brought one on their gurney.

Not all emergency services carry defibrillators, despite their ease of use and relatively low cost. Jeff, the paramedic, was well aware that the probability of survival approaches zero if a patient in ventricular fibrillation does not get shocked within ten minutes. EMS protocols dictate that unconscious and unresponsive patients be intubated as quickly as possible—requiring the insertion of an airway pipe into the patient's throat so that oxygen can be forced into the lungs. Cardiac arrest patients also require special drugs to help the blood flow into the major organs—neurological damage was highly likely without the oxygen and drugs. All of this was vital, but only if they could get Carolyn's heart beating again.

The second EMT was busy preparing the LIFEPAK®12 Defibrillator/Monitor, and he pulled out two disposable patch electrodes ready to attach to Carolyn's chest. The team had been in this situation close to a hundred times over the previous five years, and yet they had been successful in saving just one patient. Could this be their second miracle save?

Exhausted, and now no longer needed, Tom decided he didn't want witness any more of the emergency. He needed to get away before he heard any bad news; he sensed that the ominous third option he feared was not far away.

Standing nearby, Jim was trying to focus on Kathy, as she briefed the EMTs, but out of the corner of his eye he had seen them prepare the needles, and take out the paddles. He couldn't bear to see them stick things into Carolyn. He felt empty and emotionally exhausted. He turned and walked away, thinking, "I've done all I can." But he didn't think it was enough. He was preparing himself for her demise. After all, he had seen her fade away, right there in his hands.

࿔

Bruce was relieved to see the EMTs rush in and attend to Carolyn. Having seen medical emergencies depicted on TV, he was surprised how different the real event was in front of him. The door was still open and he was shocked to see them preparing to cut Carolyn's blouse off. He turned away, unable to witness her privacy being invaded.

"I don't think they will be able to save her. It has been too long," Bruce felt certain of these thoughts. He wanted to trust and have hope, but he suspected the worst. "She has been blue for a long time now. She hadn't responded to any of their actions."

Bruce turned as Jim staggered out of the room, and saw the vacant look in his eyes. At that moment Bruce realized they had yet another difficult task, "Oh my god, we have to tell her husband."

❧

As soon as the EMTs were ready, the paramedic stopped squeezing the BVM bag, and performed the endoctracheal intubation to secure an open airway, using a seven-point-five millimeter tube. They connected the oxygen cylinder with the regulator set to deliver twenty-five liters of oxygen per minute. Using a stethoscope, Jeff checked that Carolyn's breath sounds were clear and normal, indicating the tube was in the right place—not in her stomach, or in just one lung. That took care of the airway and oxygen, but they still had to get her heart beating again.

They needed to connect the defibrillator. The EMT placed a sticky patch electrode on Carolyn's ribs below her left breast, another higher up on her right side and clipped on the leads. The large display on the cardiac monitor sprang to life, and immediately showed a chaotic squiggle with no recognizable rhythm. A tinny mechanical voice emanated from the unit, announcing that this was a "shockable rhythm".

But the EMTs had beaten the unit to the diagnosis and were already following the cardiac arrest/V-fib protocol. They were working in unison, a well-oiled machine, and had wasted no time. All three of them had watched the monitor, and seen the telltale signs of ventricular fibrillation—random, unrelated waves.

Carolyn needed to be shocked immediately; before they did anything else, since the amount of energy needed to convert VF rapidly increases with time.

"I'm clear, are you clear?" The paramedic checked that no one was touching Carolyn.

"We're all clear! Defibrillating at two hundred," he announced.

Carolyn's body was jolted by the charge, making her legs wriggle. The monitor showed her vitals were still sporadic after the first shock, and she reverted to V-fib again. The chaotic squiggle that returned after the big spike showed that her heart muscle was not responding to the shocks.

"Epinephrine 1:10,000 IV push."

The paramedic inserted an eighteen gauge intravenous line into Carolyn's right jugular vein, and pushed the syringe full of adrenaline hormone into the IV followed by a liter of normal saline to flush the drug through her blood vessels. It would also boost the fluids in her system to increase her blood pressure.

The monitor still showed VF.

They had to shock her a second time. Then a third, this time at a higher energy setting, but it was not successful.

It was time to try more drugs, but the paramedic could not use epinephrine again, as it is less effective a second time.

"Three hundred milligrams Cordarone."

He waited a few moments for the drug to circulate, and administered another shock, with nearly twice the energy level as previously.

"Sinus tachycardia."

Carolyn had converted to a regular rhythm, but an abnormally fast one, so the paramedic watched the monitor carefully for Ventricular Tachycardia. This dangerously fast heartbeat often precedes V-fib.

It did not appear.

"Time to get her out of here," the paramedic said quietly to the two EMTs, "her pupils are not reacting normally. I don't know the cause, she could have an aneurysm."

They said nothing in reply, but quickly completed the protocol. The three of them had been working for nineteen minutes and eventually gotten her heart to beat regularly again, but she had been down for over twelve minutes before that. More than half an hour without a pulse!

In preparation for the trip to the emergency ward, Carolyn was given 100mg Lidocaine bolus to suppress the electrical disturbance in her cardiac tissues. This would reduce the chance of her arresting again during transport, but they did not remove the defibrillator. She was highly unstable and they could not afford any delay if she did revert.

❧

Tom had seen the apprehensive look on the faces in the corridor when he walked out of the room, but he could not voice his fears. Instead, he looked away and decided to wash his face and clear his mind of the horror. He had to wipe the sweat out of his eyes as he walked down the hall to the bathroom. Once inside, alone and seeing his reflection in the mirror, Tom could no longer ignore his misgivings; "Even if she lives, we will not know about her brain for quite a while." He feared the worst; surely she had suffered some damage. How could he live with it? "Wouldn't it be better if…." He closed his eyes.

❧

Randy couldn't stop thinking about that tragic time in 1984 when he and the nurse couldn't save the guy. Standing by himself just outside the conference room, he was feeling emotionally numb and dazed; he was at a loss what to do. Several people came toward him, as they knew he had been doing the CPR and they started asking questions.

"How did she look?"

"Did you ever hear her heartbeat?"

Randy saw tears in their eyes, and he could hear somebody nearby praying out loud. They wanted to know what had happened behind the closed door. They were thinking he had saved Carolyn's life.

"I'm no hero," he told them, "Honestly, the only thing that might save her is those EMTs and their 'jump-start' cables." He paused, and then closed the conversation with, "She didn't look any good." Randy wished he could have done more for them—and Carolyn. "What can I say," he thought, "I don't know if she is gonna be all right or not. And I've no answers for them."

Several people started to describe similar situations they had experienced, and asked him if this was the same, but Randy could only reply, "I don't know."

He just didn't want to get into the speculation that inevitably follows a calamity. And he certainly didn't want to talk about that last time, nearly twenty years earlier.

※

Now that his role in the emergency was "over", Jim had a further duty to consider. He agreed with Bruce, "We have to get to Jeremy." They both went in search of a private phone, aware that only one of them had ever spoken to Carolyn's husband before.

In his regular conversations with Carolyn, Jim remembered how she had talked about her Australian spouse with such pride and joy. He knew that this phone call to Boston was going to be difficult. We had never met, but from the way Carolyn had spoken so highly of me, Jim was not at all prepared for my odd response. It was as though I did not realize how much danger Carolyn was in. Jim hadn't wanted to be alarmist so he had skipped the graphic details of Carolyn's collapse. But he could hardly believe those words emanating from the earpiece.

My reply, "Oh, she'll be okay," just wasn't the right response!

Jim wanted to look me in the eye and say, "No Jeremy, she didn't just pass out here. This is really serious." But that was not possible and he needed to find another way. He knew I should immediately "come on down to Dallas", but he wasn't hearing that from me.

"Why is he unsure about this? I have described pretty much what has happened to her," Jim wondered. "I don't think Jeremy understands. I'm not getting through to him. Maybe it's just that Aussie laid back attitude. How much more can I say? I don't want to scare him, but he needs to know how important this is. He can't be thinking that he'll just check back with us a bit later on. She may not survive this."

※

When the EMTs finally opened the conference room door, Mark expected to see a white sheet over a body; it had been such a long time. He couldn't bear to look. He had seen the look of failure on each of Tom, Randy and Jim's faces as they had left the room.

The paramedic rushed out with Carolyn strapped to the gurney. There was an oxygen bottle attached to a tube in her mouth and an IV in her neck. While she did not appear as lifeless as Mark had feared, she didn't seem any better than when the emergency team had arrived over twenty minutes ago.

As the EMTs pushed the gurney down the corridor, Sara could see the cardiac monitor propped up between Carolyn's legs. The sight of a heartbeat on the large LCD screen filled Sara with hope.

They wheeled Carolyn past Randy and Dave Wylie, another executive from Jim's team. Carolyn's eyes were closed, her lips were blue, the patches and leads were still connected, and they were in a hurry.

"She don't look too good," Dave said.

"She doesn't look good at all," Randy agreed.

Randy felt a heavy depression come over him. "She is not going to make it," he thought. "When I was a policeman I didn't know any of them, and it didn't hit me at all," he recalled. "But this time I'm connected to her; we talk all the time." Looking for an explanation for his despondent feelings he reflected, "It isn't part of this job to experience an emergency like this."

The ambulance siren echoed down the hall; Carolyn and the emergency services team were gone. The room seemed so empty and abandoned, only the debris remained; plastic caps, tubes and wrappings scattered all over the floor, and the tables and chairs piled up in one corner.

"What do we do now?" Mark wondered. There was a vacuum, an anti-climax, and they were adrift emotionally, needing some direction.

Sarah gathered everyone together and gave everybody an opportunity to express their shock, and then she asked if they should continue the course, cancel it, or reconvene later. Her words touched Mark, and he looked around the group to gauge their reactions. There were only a few who knew exactly what they wanted, and they were not shy in expressing their thoughts.

Pam, Bruce and Karen had just one thing to say, "We want her back." They were genuinely concerned and wanted to deal with the loss in their own way.

Randy did not want to go back in there—where it had happened; it was too soon. He wanted to be alone.

Kathy had returned to her nurses' convention meeting, and Tom was nowhere to be seen.

Consensus was easily reached; they would reconvene later in the day to decide.

~

Having seen the ambulance leave with Carolyn on board, Karen wanted to follow. Bruce agreed, as he felt compelled to follow his conscience. "I'm not staying here, I'm absolutely going to the hospital." He considered this to be the most important thing to do. "If they try to stop me I'll tell them, 'I don't care if I lose my job, you're not going to make me stay here. Carolyn is not going to be alone,' and I know that Pam and Karen are right with me on this."

They asked the hotel staff where the hospital was and the best way to get there. The hotel shuttle bus was immediately offered, with a driver who knew the route. Was there anything else they could do?

Pam also could not have Carolyn just leave, not like that. She and Jim climbed aboard with the other two. Karen was surprised to learn that the driver was a medical school student. She described the events to him, and asked for his interpretation. She needed an explanation. Why did this happen? He understood her need but could offer little more than some frightening medical terminology. Karen didn't ask him to elaborate.

All three of them were in the bus sitting next to Jim, who was busy on his cell phone. Karen realized that she didn't really know Jim, who was two management levels above her, and yet they were all sharing this harrowing experience. There was a bond building between them. "We have to look after Carolyn" didn't need to be said. Her instinct was to collaborate and "solve the problem". She knew that Bruce and Jim were arranging transportation for Carolyn's husband, and she hoped he could get there soon. "We should be with her until Jeremy gets here," she said to Bruce.

Pam and Karen recognized that Jim's priority was clear: "Carolyn is more important than anything else right now," was written all over his face. She was part of the family, and they realized that their company had a human side to it, something that had never before been revealed so clearly. It was touching and impressive. This was a whole new perspective for the three managers, as they adjusted to the shock and suddenness of Carolyn's collapse.

"How was it possible for us not to notice this compassion and care within the company before?" Karen wondered in silence.

All of them had been deeply touched by the tragic event. And yet it was uncommon to perceive such a significant human expression from the bureaucratic monolith. It created a strong feeling of loyalty to be part of this "IBM family".

Baylor Medical Center was less than five miles down the road, and the EMTs had already wheeled Carolyn into the ER by the time Jim and the three managers arrived. Carolyn was lying on a gurney at the back of the emergency room, surrounded by a sea of green bodies as the doctors assessed her condition. Karen clearly saw the medical staff buzzing around Carolyn as if she was a queen bee in the hive. A series of blood tests were required without delay; the orders barked staccato: "CBC, CMP, CPK, CK-MB, ABG." The emergency care specialist needed to know more than the EMTs could tell him, and wanted to check for the enzymes and proteins that indicate heart muscle damage. He also needed to measure Carolyn's arterial blood gas to determine the oxygen level. Only then would they be able to determine the next course of action.

Suddenly, the medical team started working on Carolyn furiously.

"She must have relapsed," Karen thought, as she saw them doing more CPR, stringing up extra IV lines and zapping Carolyn, again and again and again. Then the curtain was closed. Karen could no longer see the struggle for life, but she did hear the frightening sounds.

The ER waiting room was not a calm place, with a lot of activity and complaints from people with injuries, and the admitting nurse could see how distraught Pam and Karen were. She sensed that Carolyn's workmates needed some time-out to adjust to the shock of her cardiac arrest, and suggested the hospital chapel might be a more suitable place than the ER. She led them down the hall only to find the chapel was occupied—a bereaved family had just been told that a loved one had passed away.

The hospital Chaplain had seen the managers outside the occupied chapel and recognizing their grief, offered to sit with them in the ER waiting room. Pam didn't know how to handle the trauma, and it showed. The Chaplin decided to unlock a doctor's office and let the three managers comfort each other in private—a very generous and trusting thing to do—and Pam appreciated the gesture. There was little for the three of them to do anyway. The medical staff had their protocols to follow, and a battery of tests to perform on Carolyn, before they would have any news.

໖

Several hours had passed and yet there was no word as to Carolyn's condition. Jim did not want to leave the hospital, and felt responsible for Carolyn until Jeremy arrived. He felt uncomfortable with inactivity, and being from Atlanta, he was unsure of the hospital's standing. He wondered if she was getting the best care. The doctor who spoke to Jeremy had uttered those disturbing words, "critical condition." Having had much experience with the inconsistency of medical care, Jim decided he needed to know more about the qualifications of those attending to Carolyn.

"Are these doctors any good?" he asked Mark. "Going through the ER, you don't know who you're getting," he wanted to add.

Mark, a resident of Dallas, explained that the Baylor Health System had a reputation as one of the best in the country, and that they specialized in cardiology.

Jim was immediately reassured by this, and rationalized his concern with an old family saying: "Trust God with all your heart, but don't forget to tie your own camel."

Jim still felt lost, not really knowing what was going to happen to Carolyn. She was in the doctors' hands now. He had no understanding of her medical history, no point of reference. He couldn't tell the doctors anything useful about her. He didn't even know her age.

"We will make sure Jeremy is reunited with his wife," he decided. "That, at least, is something I can help with."

❧

Sitting with the other two managers in the quiet office, Pam learned that Jim had finally gotten me to understand the gravity of the situation. "Poor guy, he must be so worried," she said under her breath. "How is he going to react when he sees Carolyn?" Pam then realized it would be many hours before I would arrive in Dallas.

A new fear emerged that Pam kept to herself. She was now worried that Carolyn might die there, alone. What should they do?

Pam remembered seeing a gift shop on the way in to the emergency ward. She decided there was something she could do, "I have to get an angel to watch over her." The choice was porcelain or silver. Karen had come along to help out. They couldn't decide which one, and bought both.

❧

David Spofford, Carolyn's business analyst, was holding the fort at the office in Boston. He was proud to have been asked to monitor the Business Unit's activities while Carolyn and her three managers were attending the course in Dallas. Carolyn had inspired him to seek a leadership role in the company, and he saw this as a chance to show how capable and competent he was. Sure, it was a small thing; but they had asked *him,* ahead of the more experienced staff. He saw it as an opportunity to rise to the challenge.

It was mid afternoon in Boston, when David got a call from someone he hardly ever spoke to, asking what had happened to Carolyn, wanting to know if she was all right. David had no idea what this person was talking about and said so. But he was puzzled about the caller's question, so abruptly asking about Carolyn. A minute later a female colleague from another floor came into his office and said, "I heard that Carolyn has collapsed." She, too, asked if David knew what had happened to Carolyn. David was now worried. What had these people heard? What was going on?

His thoughts were interrupted by a call from Bruce Senecal in Dallas, who had some details, but no explanation. "Carolyn has collapsed, maybe a heart attack. She stopped breathing. They have her on life support. Please pray for her, we don't know what is going to happen." David was stunned and shocked to hear that his boss was in danger; she didn't look to him to be a candidate for a heart attack. She wasn't old, wasn't overweight, and didn't smoke; in fact she was always so full of life. He had been impressed with Carolyn's energy and enthusiasm for their new mission, and felt she was making great progress in leading the team through a difficult organizational transition.

David sensed this to be a turning point in his aspirations. He saw it as an excellent opportunity for him to demonstrate his own leadership abilities. He was not so vain as to think it would be noticed or have an immediate impact, but it was going to be a fraught few days until they knew what had happened. He was also eager to see how well he would operate in a crisis, to see how his military peacekeeping experience in Bosnia might apply to the corporate world. He gathered everyone together to make the announcement. It was the first time David had addressed all of Carolyn's team, and what he had to say was very difficult to deliver calmly. He didn't want to alarm anyone, but he felt that they ought to be told immediately. He was unsure what to say and thought, "We have just started to get to know her, and there is so much hope for the future, how do I tell them? They are going to be shocked and upset for such a dramatic event like this to come out of the blue."

He repeated what little news he had been given, and asked everyone to pray for Carolyn.

"Oh my God, what does this mean?" he heard someone say. They were searching for details or answers, and yet he knew virtually nothing about Carolyn's situation. He shared the uncertainty and fear they were feeling. Everyone was concerned for Carolyn, and there was a stunned silence as they moved off to their own spaces to digest the awful news. David was glad he didn't have many details to relay, as he knew there would have been tears if he had.

David planned on keeping everyone informed, hoping the team would try to carry on as best they could; he definitely didn't want them to be left leaderless. He was looking to give them some assuredness, wanting to help them remain calm and not to panic. They all loved Carolyn and were obviously worried. He could almost hear them say, "She was walking us through this big change, what will this mean to us?" What indeed. Bruce had not been positive in his tone or manner, and David feared that Carolyn was not coming back at all.

Sitting in his office, trying to focus on the regular tasks he had to deal with that day, David could not avoid confronting his own mortality. Still in his early thirties, it was not a familiar topic, but he did start checking off in his mind all the things he could do to improve his health and lifestyle. He couldn't get over how things can change instantly and without warning. He wondered where he would be on his deathbed, and how it would happen. He knew that this was a normal reaction to such a catastrophe, but it still seemed morbid.

❧

By mid afternoon, Dallas time, Jim Hardee was worried. He was relieved that I was now on my way, but also terrified that Carolyn would die before I arrived. He had to focus all his spiritual energy on Carolyn. "She is in the hands of God now, her family must be supported. We must do everything we can to help them," he told himself over and over.

Carolyn's collapse had hit Jim very hard. To him, she was a very special, unique person. He had hundreds of people in his charge, and as Vice President there were serious and complex issues to resolve every day. Of all his experiences in life so far, this was the most difficult—

even more traumatic than the loss of his father. This time he was a participant in the tragedy, not a spectator. He had actually seen the life in Carolyn's eyes dissolve as he held her.

"She's gone," he thought.

One doesn't have to deal with that very often in life. Jim felt helpless and lost. Everyone had been doing everything they possibly could, but it did not seem to be enough to bring Carolyn back to life.

Sitting in the ER waiting room with nothing to do but wait, Jim could not stop the ominous thoughts, as he really didn't hold out much hope for Carolyn.

"She's on life support, chances are she's not coming back," he reasoned. He did not discuss these thoughts.

❧

Leaving Jim and the three managers at the hospital to keep vigil over Carolyn, Mark Johnson returned to the hotel to seek out Randy Fitch. He had a mission; some questions needed answers.

"The doctors would like to know if she had a certain look on her face, like a gasping look about her? Did she clench her teeth?" he asked.

But Randy couldn't remember any details. Even though the emergency occurred only a short while earlier, the events were all a blur for him.

Mark passed on what little he knew about Carolyn's condition. Hardly anything of substance, but it had been hours now, and so it was good news that she was still alive.

Relived to find out that Carolyn had survived, Randy wanted to let Tom O'Brien know. He hadn't seen him since the episode, and didn't even know which hotel room Tom was in. He had to ask the hotel operator to connect them.

"Tom, this is Randy. She's alive!" Randy cried into the phone. The call was short. He could sense there was relief, but Tom hadn't seemed to know what to say.

"He is in a dark place; disconnecting from it all," Randy thought.

"I'm glad I called to tell him, as he needs to know that Carolyn has survived."

But Tom had not shared his fear that just surviving could possibly be the worst outcome. He almost felt responsible, and couldn't face the ramifications. He really couldn't bear to know.

Randy had also wanted to go to the hospital and see Carolyn, but he knew that she would be in intensive care. He expected only family members would be allowed to visit. He also thought this was probably a good thing as he didn't want to do something embarrassing like break down in front of her. Although he wanted to see Carolyn for himself, he would have to trust that she was going to be all right.

Randy mentally summed up his actions and put the matter to rest, "All that pumping, and all that blowing, it was truly for nothing. Only those paddles could save her."

Chapter 2

WELCOME TO DALLAS

*The single biggest problem in communication
is the illusion that it has taken place.*

—George Bernard Shaw

I will always remember my forty-second birthday, for that was the day that Carolyn and I were married. There was no indication that a scant six weeks later she would be the victim of a sudden cardiac arrest. Carolyn had been enthusiastic about her new position as an executive of that well-known multinational corporation, but not necessarily happy about being sent to Texas for a conference so soon after our wedding. She would have preferred some time for us to settle in and adjust to our new routines. In just two months we had packed up our furniture and most of our belongings to put into storage, traveled half way across the world, moved into a strange new home, gotten married and now we suddenly faced a serious medical emergency.

As I was sitting on the floor that fateful Thursday morning, hearing those terrifying words "critical condition" emanate from the phone, I desperately tried to connect them to my world. I was not aware of the details, but I knew that something dreadful had happened to Carolyn in Dallas, and I was not there. What should I do? What had happened to her? I like to be in control of my domain, but this situation was clearly outside my zone of influence. How could this be? I was stunned and disbelieving, surely it was not true?

I'd had only a minute or two to comprehend the enormity of Jim's words, and I did not know that he had witnessed the tragic event.

Despite the doctor's frightful words, I could not accept that

Carolyn was in danger, especially as we had spoken only a short while earlier and she seemed fine. Neither Jim nor I were able to overcome the confusion, but he had the composure to consider my position; I was new to the country, my wife was away on business and I was now told to "get on down here" as Carolyn was seriously ill—maybe even to handle the onerous responsibilities as her "next of kin".

I was mentally numb and could not think what to do or say, but the next thing I heard Jim say eased my overwhelming panic.

"Don't worry about the travel arrangements, I'll have my assistant call you with the details, and we'll get you down here as fast as we can," he said with an ease that belied his true feelings.

Incredibly, that simple statement brought me enormous relief, and the microcosm of my life started to feel under control again. Of course I could fly on down to Texas at a moment's notice. Yeah, I could do that, no problemo. I'm a very task oriented person and here was a task on which I could focus my mind, dispelling the turmoil for a few moments. What time was the next flight? I'll just pack a few things, it's all coming back to me now, like second nature: toiletries, suit-pack, smalls and shoes. What shirts to take? What's the weather like in Dallas—hot isn't it? What did Carolyn pack yesterday?

Uh-oh, how long will I be there? What am I going to Dallas for? Oh, that's right. I'd better bring some clothes for Carolyn, nice comfy ones for the trip home. That's what I'm doing; I'm bringing her home. These thoughts were comforting, and a false sense of control and normalcy returned.

As I packed some of her underwear, dressing gown and slippers, I considered taking a camera to take her photo. I cannot say there was a great deal of thought in the action, and I could not have known what I was going to capture, but it could be the last image I had of her—not exactly a memento, more a definitive symbol of the reality. A reality I had not yet acknowledged. Did not the Native Americans believe that a camera could capture the spirit? I wanted more than that, and intended to bring her home, and if not, then I needed a last picture of her. Why was I thinking like this? Maybe it was just the Boy Scout in me coming out—be prepared.

The next two hours flew past in a blur of phone calls on both phones as I dashed from one room to the next, packing and panicking. The first call was to my mother-in-law, Helen Lema. No answer. Next I tried Carolyn's brother David. How should I break the news? What news? I didn't know what was wrong with Carolyn. What would I say to him?

Dave took the devastating report well, probably due to his training as a counselor and long involvement in dealing with crises, but he was clearly shocked. His next few words, however, raised a new dilemma, one I had not expected.

"I'll come with you to Dallas," he said.

"Oh, I don't think you need to do that," I stammered, hoping he was merely offering to come. I was barely able to cope with my own travel arrangements, let alone think about a companion. I reconsidered the situation. What right did I have to tell Carolyn's sibling that he needn't be there!

The silence on the line told me I could have handled the reply better.

My brother-in-law is broad and stocky, solid and dark, with a hard penetrating stare. I see him as swarthy and streetwise, but he is also wonderfully gentle and kind, and always polite. It's just that he resembles a Hell's Angel; that long ponytail down his back, Harley Davidson motorcycle, leather vest, and deep, gruff voice. I started thinking that if he wanted to come with me, by all means, he had a right to. I wouldn't argue.

Dave continued as though he hadn't heard my faux pas. He asked me what flight I was taking. But I didn't know! I was in Boston, and he was in Providence, Rhode Island. How would these arrangements work? He said he'd find out and call me back.

A few minutes after the call ended, I realized that I was pleased that Dave's suggestion had forced me to confront my natural tendency to be independent. Being an only child, I am very used to doing things my own way. In fact, sometimes, I prefer to do everything on my own, even to the point of resenting the help of well-intentioned people. On this occasion, I felt relieved. It was dawning on me that I might need some support.

Another phone call ended this reverie, forcing me to confront the reality that I had yet to break the news to Carolyn's mother, Helen. I was somewhat better at handling the situation now that I had actually said the words aloud.

"Carolyn has been admitted to hospital in Dallas. She has had a cardiac arrest, but she's going to be all right," I told Helen. I could tell that my voice sounded hesitant, and it had good reason to be. How did I know that she'd be "all right"? I was scared to admit my worst fears. I had tried to be calm and compassionate, but actually, I was panicking and feeling pessimistic.

"I'm flying down there today," I continued, filling the void at the end of the phone line. "Dave has offered to come with me. I'll call you as soon as I have more details." I'm not normally abrupt in my words. In fact, I tend to be verbose, but this was not a normal time.

I sensed that Helen hadn't fully grasped what I was saying, but I could tell that the words "cardiac arrest" had frightened her.

"Oh no, her heart! Not another one, not my Carolyn. How could this happen to her, too?" Helen said to herself more than to me. Five of her brothers had died at an early age from heart related illness, and about ten years earlier Carolyn's father was found dead at the wheel of his car, from a presumed heart attack, on his way to golf. This was alarming for Helen—the son-in-law from "down under" breezing into her world and now calling to say her youngest daughter was at death's door. What else could I say? This was a totally foreign situation for me, in more ways than one!

I couldn't think of anything else to say to Helen's comment. She seemed to be resigned to the fact that Carolyn was lost, and yet she couldn't face another death. She obviously wanted to be with Carolyn but realized that she was not in a position to fly to Dallas, and so she could only pray for her. We said goodbye hurriedly before either of us could break down. I repeated that I would call her when I had further details. I also assumed that Dave would soon talk to Helen in person, which was what she really needed.

"God Bless" was her reply. I had always found faith to be a perplexing thing, but I was starting to realize the real and valuable place it can occupy in our lives.

The phone rang again and this time it was Jim's assistant, Vicki Cook, calling from Atlanta to say that Carolyn's assistant, Jean Irwin, in Boston, had all my travel arrangements organized. Vicki said that Jean would call me soon with the details. I was struggling to keep up with all the names and places, and a sense of helplessness crept in. Vicki apologized to me for the situation, (as if it was her fault!) and asked if I needed anything. I confessed that I had no idea where I was going in Dallas, nor how I would get there. She calmly gave me Jim's cell number and told me that one of Carolyn's staff would meet me at the airport in Dallas. I was touched by the closeness of her tone and the words she used. I started to get an inkling of the power a large organization can wield when a real emergency occurs. How often we complain about those artificial emergencies created by bureaucracy and deadlines, that seemingly can't be resolved, but in this case nothing was a problem.

My mind continued this thought in the background, as I recalled the incredible acts of rescue and recovery following the devastating September 11th attacks the year before. We all have such a capacity for selfless contribution in times of catastrophe, coping with immediate needs, making things seem under control and effective when that is usually the furthest from the truth. Would we be able to return to a normal life, or was this the end?

I could not stop thinking that Carolyn had had an aneurism and would not recover. What would I do? We had only just arrived in this country, and it was wonderful learning new things, finding our way.

But now, a disaster I was not equipped to handle, threatened to ruin it all. I put these thoughts away. They weren't helping me deal with the matters at hand and I had no real understanding of what had happened to her anyway.

Dave called back to say the next available flight cost over twelve hundred dollars, which he couldn't afford. He wanted to be on the same flight as me, to help me through this emergency, and I considered offering to pay with our credit card, but realized that could be complicated. He wanted to help, not to make things harder. I told him I'd be okay on my own, as the company had some fantastic people looking after all the travel logistics. Dave apologized for not being able to join me, and said he would look into alternatives. He wished me well.

The anguish flooded back again. Must try to think only of the tasks before me. Must be ready for the car to get me to Logan airport on time. Got to get the fax from the office downstairs for the plane tickets. Thank goodness we don't have any pets. What have I forgotten? Can't deal with eating right now, I'll give lunch a miss. These disjointed thoughts were all I could manage, just holding my head above water, but remarkably I hadn't broken down—yet.

Suddenly there was nothing for me to do but wait. Traveling is always a case of hurry up and wait. Surges of activity, followed by endless periods of nothing; someone else's schedule, you have to fit into their timetable, they decide when—not you.

The muscles in my face felt as solid as concrete from the tension in my clenched jaw, as I continued worrying about the sudden change to our future. No matter how much I wanted to ignore it, I could not stop the harsh reality. I was on my own, something disastrous had occurred to the love of my life, and she needed me by her side. We had spoken at seven o'clock that morning and she was in perfect health then. How did this terrible thing happen? What possible reason could there be for her to be struck down so suddenly? There had been no accident, she was safe inside a hotel conference room, she was among people she knew, and she was coming home the next day. How could that have changed?

Carolyn didn't like going away on trips without me. Funny how things change, I remember her stories about living in Perth, Australia, when she longed for the escape that her business trips to the Pilbara provided. Those trips were not what I would call fun; thousands of miles from home, out in the desert; tiny little towns established just to support the mining operations, dusty and hot, coarse humor and nothing to do in the off-hours. At that time she was unhappy at home and fleeing to anywhere else was desirable.

So there I was, also preparing to fly out to a remote, hot and dusty part of my new country, not quite the desert, but very nearly. And it was not desirable for me. This was no escape; I was heading *towards* my dread, not away from it.

As I got my things together and went downstairs to meet the driver, I searched for a reason for this mishap. Surely it couldn't be any more than that; possibly it was a dreadful mistake. Was this one of the responsibilities of marriage? "In sickness and in health, for richer or poorer." I had never faced death before, and had previously felt equipped to handle the disasters life threw at me. But this time I was definitely outside my comfort zone, and more than a little spaced out from the enormity of the situation.

Moving from front porch to back seat, I felt like a piece of luggage. The polished, black Lincoln Town Car was big like a hearse and, gazing vacantly out the window, I vaguely recognized the route to the airport. Not so many weeks earlier, I had arrived via these same roads and highways. The driver attempted some small talk. I knew I needed to respond, if only to acknowledge my existence in his domain.

"My wife's had a cardiac arrest, and I'm going to Dallas to collect her," I murmured.

The car suddenly became very quiet, although I was comfortable with that. It was not his fault. I was only just coping with the shock and had no powers of concentration at all. I hardly knew what was happening around me, so paralyzing were my thoughts and fears.

I had to test out the reactions to my new truth, and that statement: "My wife has had a sudden cardiac arrest." How did it sound? What did he think? What did I think? What did that matter? What can I do to stop these morbid thoughts?

We stopped; I looked up and had no idea where I was. The driver assured me this was the terminal I needed. How did he know? Did Jean tell him? The building looked totally unfamiliar to me, but he had placed my bags on the curb and was ready to drive off, so I picked them up and wandered inside. As I entered the terminal, I realized that he must have already been paid.

Departures at Logan airport was a madhouse with people hustling and bustling everywhere, while others, like me, merely stood still, looking lost and bewildered. Uniformed gatekeepers were mustering the passengers, picking on one here, one there, checking the flight number and insisting that they have their bags with them at all times. The scene reminded me of shearing time at my grandfather's farm and his sheep dog, Trigger, who every now and then, would nip the heels of an errant ewe, just so the rest of the flock didn't get any ideas of not following the corrals into the shearing shed. And, just like sheep, we all obeyed the airport gatekeepers. There was a long line of passengers checking in to American Airlines, and I staggered along with the tide as it ebbed and flowed towards the counter.

The barrage of fears began again. Oh no, this queue is too long. I'll never make the flight. I'm booked on the 4pm as well. I have to remember to call Jean if I make it—she was most insistent on that. I was sure everyone could see the anxiety on my face. In a panic, I realized I only had a faxed e-Ticket receipt. Where do I get the airline ticket? It was so unlike my pre 9/11 Australian business trips, that I wasn't sure I could cope. After an indeterminate period of time, I was shepherded to the next available check-in counter, where the clerk looked at me in a detached way as I handed over the fax copy of the e-Ticket.

"What flight?" was all he said to me.

"Er, Dallas. I only have an e-Ticket, is that OK?" I asked, fumbling my words. I also handed over my only photo ID, an Australian driver's license, while he started typing for what seemed a disturbingly long time. Oh, please, let there be no problem.

He looked up at me with a bemused expression, "Just that bag?"

I had packed my standard business-travel suit-pack. Somehow, it felt more comfortable and familiar than a suitcase. I had thought of carrying it onboard to save time, but the look on his face unnerved me. I asked if I needed to check it in. His reply didn't help.

"Looks okay to me, but you wouldn't want to have it rejected at the gate." He then raised an eyebrow, and looked at me expectantly.

So many decisions! I accepted his cryptic advice, and checked in the bag. But then I scrambled to take out the things I needed on board. He handed over my boarding pass and I noticed it was a first class seat; I had been standing in the wrong line! There was no one waiting at first class check-in—no wonder he had given me those perplexing looks. Ever the critical perfectionist, I was judging myself, but then, I realized it didn't matter, and willed myself to relax and focus on the important stuff. "Carolyn needs you to be calm and collected," I reminded myself.

Security was another hurdle to overcome. First we were screened at the terminal entrance and then again at the gate, and of course, I was singled out for a full search. Luckily, I had checked my bag after all. Shoes off, coat on the table, standing like a crucifix while they waved their magic wand about and pronounced me safe. I was allowed to board the plane.

I had just a few moments to ring Jean and tell her I was on the earlier flight and to cancel the later booking. When I told her that I must have been bumped up a grade as I got a first class seat, she just said, "I know" and wished me good luck. I noticed a great deal of compassion in her voice, and hoped she was being more pessimistic than was needed. I was disturbed by how unaware I was of simple details like the class of ticket I had, and wondered how I was going to cope with the difficult stuff in Dallas. Did Jean tell me I was flying first class? What did it matter anyway? I'd be on the plane soon, and have that waiting thing to do again.

Finally, I was able sit down, and decided to just let the anxiety take its course. As I closed my eyes, a wave of fear passed through me, and made me shudder. I blinked a couple of times. The dreaded thoughts would not stop. What could have happened to her? Is she going to recover? I was so scared she would end up in a coma. How would I tell her mother? What if Carolyn doesn't make it? What will I do? Would I be able to stay in the country? What about the green card application? And what about the apartment rental-contract that we had just signed? My world was crashing down around me. I felt helpless.

❧

I was leaving Salem, where we lived on Boston's North Shore, at an especially picturesque time. October is when the spectacular fall colors reign. Autumn in New England endeavors to capture the last vestiges of the summer fire, before the cold, hard north wind blows the fragile dying leaves off their branches in retribution. Summer has gone, and there are no more spent hurricanes seasoning the town with Floridian humidity. The sun struggles to prevail, but it is a tepid little affair that doesn't last beyond the business hours. Those languid rays serve as a beacon to guide us through the snow that envelops the trees, smothering the streets and silencing the raucousness of Halloween. Winter seems to last longest, and nobody wants summer to end. Spring shoots by, but fall is never forgotten.

My first experience of a New England fall was in November, 2000. I had been on a tour of IT establishments in Massachusetts. Flying into Boston that cloudless afternoon I had my face pressed against the glass, in awe of the spectacular colors. Surely it's not possible for the trees to be more vibrant than gaudy calendars and postcards? The leaves were so brilliant; red and yellow, almost clashing with the brown trunks and tinges of green, like a book of matches struck all at once.

I did not see any "trees on fire" on that flight to Dallas. My view on the world had closed in—I was in shock. Time stood still, and then, like a scratched DVD, it would skip forward, and I had to catch up. I did not look out the window after take off; I did not look at anything until the flight attendant suddenly appeared before me.

"Would you like something to drink before lunch, sir?" I gazed up, and managed to put on a veil of normalcy, pushing the thoughts and fears aside; they were not helping me. "Take little baby steps to your destination Jeremy," I said to myself silently. "One thing at a time, one task after another. You can cope that way."

The woman in the seat next to me started some small talk. She was in the Telecommunications industry, and I avoided my morbid thoughts by listening to her reason for travel, what her job was and other distracting details. Funny how these things are so relevant and important in normal circumstances; I had never appreciated the difference before. I half-heartedly explored what position she had, where she was located, and what she was doing in Boston. I was considering whether she could be a good contact for me, since I was looking for employment prospects while waiting for that all-important green card.

It was a long flight, and *The Importance of Being Earnest* was showing. I'd had a couple of strong drinks, and felt much calmer, though not merry. I found the tension oozing out of me, and managed to laugh often and a little maniacally, at the hilarious predicaments Oscar Wilde had created for the characters, despite having seen the very same movie a few months earlier in Australia.

My escape into the headphones dissolved with the clouds outside, as I arrived into Dallas Fort Worth airport at 7pm. Carolyn's three managers suddenly appeared before me as I followed the crowd to baggage claim. Tears threatened to flow as we hugged in one big huddle. I hadn't been touched since Carolyn had left the day before, and I needed it more than ever. It was clear by the look on their faces that Pam and Karen wanted to tell me everything, so that I could prepare for the scene at the hospital. But they refrained, as I appeared to be calm and my normal jovial self. They were expecting me to be distraught and possibly break down from the shock. Little did they know! My brave face had obviously fooled them.

"How can he be so nonchalant?" they wondered, "He must be in denial." It fit neatly with my response to Jim's phone call earlier, and confirmed in their minds that I needed a lot of support. "Good thing we are here to help him, this is going to hit him hard," they thought in unison.

Bruce took my bag, and introduced the stranger who was hovering nearby. "This is Thomas, he's going to take us straight to the hospital," I was told. "He lives here in Dallas and has a car."

Sure, okay. "Hi, Thomas," was all I could manage, but I'm sure he did not think me rude. I think he was happy just being the chauffer. I certainly wouldn't know what to say to a fellow who had just flown in to see his critically ill wife. What could a stranger say?

Leaving the airport, I was unsure of what land I was in; this one was flat and dry, just like Western Australia. "She won't like it here," I reasoned, as we headed out onto the highway. I was fairly certain I wasn't going to like it either.

There were not many minutes remaining before I had to confront my fears, and I couldn't help but reflect on where I had come from and where I was going. I was one of fifty-two million passengers emerging from the crescent terminals of DFW that year. But I was unconcerned with frequent flyer miles. I was not on business, nor was I a tourist. While my outlook was clouded with trepidation and uncertainty, it was clear in purpose. How many of those millions had their arrival so permanently preserved?

I did recall that President Kennedy had died in this city when I was a child. First, the country heard that he had been shot, just as I had first been informed that Carolyn had collapsed. Then, they were told he was dead. That was a conclusion I did not want to hear.

I could not let Dallas take my special person away, too. She was too good to die so suddenly, just as many believed JFK was. He was so popular, and eager to achieve great things in his work, just as she was. He portrayed an image of youth, health, and vigor, but hid a history of illness. Surely, Carolyn had nothing hidden.

Chapter 3

INTENSIVE CARE

Life is pleasant. Death is peaceful.
It's the transition that's troublesome.

–Isaac Asimov

The Baylor Grapevine hospital is located a couple of miles west of Dallas Fort Worth airport, south of Lake Grapevine and south-west of the cemetery. With less than two hundred beds, it was not a very large hospital, but it did have a Cardiac Diagnostic Suite and over two hundred medical staff, including specialists in Cardiac Rehabilitation.

Founded as a Christian ministry of healing in 1903, the Baylor University Medical Center originated as the Texas Baptist Memorial Sanitarium, but changed its name in 1921 to reflect the relationship with Baylor University in Waco, Texas (which is the largest Baptist University in the world). In the 1950s it was the fifth largest general hospital in the United States, and they were proud of their "hospital of tomorrow", which featured air conditioning and telephones in all patient rooms. During the Great Depression, the administrators developed the "Baylor Plan" to help the local citizens afford hospital care. It was the first pre-paid hospital insurance plan in the United States and a predecessor of Blue Cross. In 1981, the Grapevine Memorial Hospital and Clinic joined the Baylor Health Care System, and was renamed the Baylor Medical Center at Grapevine. It has since undergone the largest growth and expansion of services in its history, including adding advanced digital imaging technology, and addressed a significant need in the area—open-heart surgery.

I was not aware of these impressive details that Thursday evening in October 2002. I had very little information at all, and I was soon to find out more than I really wanted to know.

Everyone in the car was silent on the short trip from the airport, leaving me to adjust to the wretchedness I had to face. In an attempt to distract my fears, I looked out the window and noticed that the landscape was almost perfectly level, so much so, that I imagined the airport control tower would be visible from nearly every building in the area. And, apart from the shiny skyscrapers in the central business district, most of the buildings looked to be no more than four of five stories high, emphasizing how flat it was. I had no clue as to which direction we were headed, or where we were actually going, but it took less than ten minutes to get there.

As we pulled into the hospital forecourt, I felt the anxiety levels rise dramatically. Everyone had become even quieter, as though they were holding their breath. It was time for silence and motion. No words, as they might betray the illusion of normality, and pop the bubble of denial. Once inside, Bruce led the way down a brightly lit, colorless corridor.

&

Pacing up and down the ER ward had not helped Jim relax. With the three managers gone, Jim had been alone with his thoughts. Ten-hour workdays were almost routine in the office, but this day's emotional roller coaster had taken its toll. The most pressing thought, the one he couldn't resolve, the one thing he wanted to find out was, "Has Jeremy gotten to that place in his mind where he realizes that this is really serious?"

We nearly bumped into Jim at a junction of the Emergency Room corridor. He looked as though he had been up all night, his eyes were red and his hair tousled. I felt sorry for him. "This company really drives their VPs hard," was my first impression. I then realized he was as upset as I was, and I regretted the disparaging thought.

He was quick to recognize who I was, as Bruce, Pam and Karen were standing next to me. We fumbled the introductions and my task orientation kicked into gear again. I felt the need to take over the burden of attending to Carolyn, telling myself, "If I take care of it, then everything will be fine." While I knew this was totally irrational, the feeling was real and compelling.

"It's all right," I told Jim. "I'm here now. You don't have to worry."

He looked at me uncomprehendingly for a few seconds, and suggested I go to Carolyn immediately, and that we could talk later. Just before he left, he reiterated that Mark would ensure all my needs were taken care of. Without saying so, he was referring to the transportation, hotel, and those critical next-of-kin logistics that no one wanted to speak about.

We did not enter the Emergency Room where Jim had just come from. Instead, I was led towards the Intensive Care Unit (called the ICU by those acquainted with its purpose). We passed a waiting room with several people in various stages of grief. Some of them had sleeping bags and food hampers. Others were staring vacantly at the TV on the wall, the coffee cups in their hands abandoned.

We entered the ICU through large swinging doors with a push-to-release lock. A large sign on the door with red letters stipulated there was no entry for anyone other than immediate family. Inside the small cramped ward were a dozen or so cubicles, all facing the nurse's station. The first few beds were occupied. I noticed them because they had bright lights, a buzz of activity, and masses of equipment attached to the bed. We stopped outside the third one, where several nurses hovered around the bed. They suddenly stepped aside when they saw me approach.

Lying on the bed was a lifeless form with sallow skin, black and blue arms, and angry red welts just visible at the hospital gown neckline. A monitor on the wall beeped, and I saw some colored lines wiggle and the accompanying digits change. The IV stand had too many bags of liquid hanging from it, and each had a tube running into a big blue box with a keypad and an LCD display. On the other side of the bed was another machine making a regular sound, like a diaphragm going up and down. Among all of this, I saw my wife. Her hair looked familiar, as did her nose. But little else was the same.

I reached out and touched Carolyn's face; it was slack and clammy. When I leant down to kiss her cheek, my tears smeared the contact between us, intensifying the cold, lifelessness of her skin.

"I'm here darling, and everything's going to be all right," I said to her, with no possible way of knowing it to be true. I started to shake, and a moan escaped from my throat. Maybe I was telling myself that it was going to be all right—it was such a shock.

I had to be strong and capable; my poor darling was unconscious, full of tubes in every possible orifice, and pumped full of drugs. It was time for action. I needed to gain control of the situation, if only for my own preservation. Bruce was telling one of the nurses who I was, and there was a flurry of introductions. The nurse started to describe Carolyn's status. I had to pay attention, and tearing my eyes from the disastrous sight before me, I started asking questions. Why did Carolyn have those tubes down her throat, and what were the drugs in all those IV bags? What was going to happen next? Why were her arms tied down? I cannot say that I was being courteous.

I guessed the nurses were very used to those types of questions and method of delivery, because the answers came slowly and patiently, with calmness and confidence. I was told the doctor would be in soon, to tell me more.

I turned back to my darling, hoping to see some sign of life. But nothing had changed.

It was a scary sight. The harsh fluorescent light above the bed was on. She had IV tubes in her arm and her neck, each with a different colored liquid streaming into her. A clear tube ran out of her nose, and the tube in her mouth had two big, blue pipes passing over her shoulder to the large noisy ventilator machine on a stand to the left of the bed. A dozen wires connected to electrodes were stuck all over her chest and back. There was a thin, pink, rubber tube emerging from her bed covers and it disappeared under the bed. A blood pressure cuff was permanently fixed to her arm, and a strange clip like a clothes peg, with yet another a wire, covered the tip of her middle finger.

Her eyes were closed, and her head had flopped over to one side. Strangely, she looked peaceful; the worry lines on her forehead were gone and her eyelids were relaxed. Is this what death looks like? I noticed her mouth was contorted; the breathing tube had been taped to her cheek and was stretching the skin, pulling her lips back and baring her teeth. I peeled the tape back and re-stuck it so she looked more human.

I put my arms around her as best I could with all the tubes and wires. All I could manage was half a hug across her shoulders, but there was no response—just that oousst shouuw noise from the ventilator, and an unpleasant smell on her skin. From the drugs, I hoped.

I looked away, and my eyes cast about the room. No windows, no door; this was a place for serious business, and only designed for a short-term stay. On one wall there was a shelf with little figurines on it. It was a window ledge I realized, but beyond it there was the brick wall of another building abutting this one, so it hardly rated as a window. The figurines captured my attention—two angels, a tiny silver one, and one made of delicate porcelain. Where did they come from? Were they watching over her? Could it make a difference?

๛

I'm not a religious person—it had no purpose, in my mind. Darwin's natural selection fitted my engineering and science background better than stories that require faith in order to agree with them. Carolyn said I have "spirituality" within me, but I think she was describing my actions, not my beliefs. She studied many religions in her early twenties, looking for something that could comfort her both emotionally and intellectually. I wished I had that belief in a "higher power". My trust in facts and figures didn't translate so well for the dire situation she was in. Science was about to show just how ineffective and unreliable it could be when pitted against natural forces.

Before I had accepted the sight before me, Dr. Hecht introduced himself as the cardiologist, and described what he believed had happened. I could barely understand the medical jargon, and had great difficulty comprehending what he was saying.

"Her ejection fraction is twenty-five to thirty percent, the blood tests show enzymes related to heart failure, possibly cardiomyopathy, predating today's incident," he said in a matter of fact tone.

This was not sounding anything like what I had been led to expect. What about the aneurism? And what is all this about heart related problems and predating?

"Has she ever had a heart attack?" he asked me.

Only nine hours earlier I had spoken to Carolyn, and she had complained half-heartedly about having to attend the workshop, wishing she were home with me, instead. She was fine then—a healthy, fit, talking, walking, slim woman in her forties. Now, she was comatose on the bed, and a cardiologist was implying that she had a damaged heart! During her twenty years in Australia, Carolyn had been vegetarian and very careful about what she ate. She had taught me how to cook some amazing dishes; they were so clean and fresh compared to cooking with meat. She would only drink water that had been purified with reverse osmosis. I found that it, too, tasted clean and fresh; so soft and light on the tongue. I was an instant convert. Never again could I drink plain tap water. We had had a personal trainer for over twelve months, teaching us a regime of exercises and diet that would keep us in good shape for life. Carolyn was so proud to have achieved her goal of regularly running the same distance in her forties that she had done in her twenties. We pounded the streets for over three miles every morning on weekends and sometimes mid-week, too. We had both quit the cigarettes years ago. We liked a drink, but a glass of red wine over dinner was supposed to be good for your heart!

How could he be asking if she has ever had a heart attack? Old people, or those who don't look after themselves, have heart attacks.

"No, I don't think so," I mumbled. "Not in the five years we've been together. Why do you think she has had a heart attack?"

"The CT scan was normal," he looked down at the chart in his hands and flipped over a few pages. I assumed that meant they had checked her head for the suspected aneurism. "The echocardiogram shows severe systolic left ventricular dysfunction and anterior-wall hypokinesis. That is, the front part of her heart muscle is damaged and it isn't pumping adequately. Her ejection fraction is less than thirty percent, and the normal range is above fifty-five percent." He looked up and watched me intently as he continued, "It is not unusual for someone to have a small blockage that causes a heart attack and not be aware of it. Maybe a pain in the chest, like indigestion, but it could be enough to cause damage to the heart muscle."

I couldn't comprehend any of this news, and sensed they didn't know for certain what had happened—he was just guessing. My thoughts came tumbling out into the open, no longer held back in the dark recesses of my mind. I could not agree with this diagnosis. There was some mistake; she hasn't had any heart attacks!

"Also there is some concern about her lungs, specifically right upper lobe atelectasis." He saw my confusion, and paused, "Sorry, she has either a partially collapsed lung, or possibly some infiltrate."

This was all happening too fast. How could Carolyn be so sick? It must be something else. Thank God the aneurism theory had been ruled out. Could she have heart disease and not know about it? Didn't she have a check up in Australia recently? I never saw any signs, but then, her family did have a history of heart problems.

Undeterred, Dr. Hecht had little time for disbelief, and so we went through the twenty questions game. He needed to get the facts; measure, monitor, and then they could determine the cause. He had little to offer me in the way of explanation or reassurance. Pathology; Prognosis; Prescription. That's how it works. He was not uncaring. They can only deal with cold hard facts. Medicine is a science, after all.

I was left with a pile of paperwork to read, complete and sign. They would do some tests the following day. Only then would they know more. We would have to wait. In the meantime, the ICU nurses were constantly monitoring her. She was in good hands.

He would be back at seven the next morning.

∽

An ICU is not a place for healthy humans. It feels more like a place of death and despair, despite the bright lights and constant activity. There is no privacy, but the patients are hardly able to complain. Everyone is under constant critical care. They need to be visible to the nurses at all times, despite the electronic monitoring of their vital signs.

Everyone there was affected by the imminent danger the patients faced. Some patients were old and frail; others were young and critically ill. Carolyn looked the best of them all, and she had a heart that would not beat. She didn't exactly look alive, but the others looked much worse. I did not take comfort from this. She shouldn't be there at all. She couldn't have hurt her heart, and yet my heart was hurting to see her so ill.

Alone, facing the nightmare, I felt I had nothing to rely upon, no knowledge, no training, and no experience. I was surrounded by strangers in a foreign land, and a long way from home. I had just one confidante and she was comatose on the bed before me.

I stood there alone in my thoughts for quite a while before I became aware of my surroundings. There were people in the room—I could hear them murmuring behind me. There was an almost physical tension in the air. There were expectations about my reaction to what happened and what I'd been told, but none of them seemed to be positive. I took stock of the situation. Time to get back in the zone. I can take charge. I know what I have to do, not that there was much, technically, for a spouse to take care of. I am responsible for the decisions, and have the greatest capability in motivating and comforting my loved one. I know that she can beat this, and attitude is everything in this world.

My natural positive outlook finally overcame the sense of doom, and I started to interrogate the ICU nurse again, with rapid-fire questions about the drugs and the machines connected to Carolyn. I didn't mean to be nasty, and she didn't take offence. If I learned what all the equipment was for, maybe I could assimilate what was being done to help Carolyn. Without the facts, I felt lost and in the dark.

Surprisingly, I understood most of the answers, and drilled down on a few of them. I discovered that Carolyn was heavily sedated for two reasons. Firstly, her heart needed some stress-free time to recover, not only because of the enzyme indication of muscle damage, but also because it had been severely traumatized by the CPR. The nurse explained that the chest wall rubbing against the heart muscle could irritate the tissue so that it does not function properly. Secondly, and more importantly, Carolyn had been intubated, since she could not breathe on her own. It was very uncomfortable having a tube down one's throat, past the vocal chords, so most people try to pull it out if they are even slightly conscious. Therefore, sedation was required. Okay, but what if she was breathing on her own, I mused? This was something I wanted to investigate further.

The Chaplin came by to see if I wanted pastoral support; the nurses had suggested I might need it. I had no objection, but couldn't bring myself to explain my agnostic attitude. Sensing my despair, she offered to say a prayer. Rebecca's words were so poignant and touching that Pam, Karen, Bruce and I just stood stiffly around the bed, crying silently. I was amazed at her ability to touch our hearts so quickly and easily, and yet provide solace at the same time. Again, I was reminded about the power of belief.

Suddenly, it was too much for me to bear. I had to accept reality. Carolyn was near death, and there was nothing I could do about it. I broke down and sobbed. Karen put her arms around my shoulders and rubbed my back gently. It was the second time that evening that I had been embraced, and I let the emotion run its course, burying my face in her shoulder as the sobs wracked my body. Eventually, they subsided and Karen released her hold. The tension and anguish had dissipated. I stood up straight, wiped my eyes and thanked her.

Soon afterwards, I was left alone with Carolyn; just the two of us and the blinking, beeping, sucking machines. I considered my little girl a fighter; strong willed and powerful. She wouldn't let anything stop her from achieving her goals, and I didn't think she'd give up on this one either. After all, they had tied her down hadn't they? Karen had seen my wife sit bolt upright in the emergency room at one stage, causing a stir among the nurses. I gathered that this was normal behavior for someone who is intubated, and that the restraints were for her protection. It was important that she did not pull out the endoctracheal tube in her throat, as it has a small balloon on the end to keep it in place and seal the airway. She could damage her vocal chords if it was not removed correctly.

The mechanical ventilator and oxygen supply were keeping Carolyn's blood oxygen level high, and the drugs were helping her heart recover, plus she was paralyzed so that her body's natural mechanisms could cope with the damage. "Paralyzed" was how the doctors described it to me, although I preferred the nurses' term, "sedated". So much easier to accept, so less permanent, a more deliberate word—something that could be undone.

Looking down at Carolyn on the bed, so still and unresponsive, I had to accept their reasoning. It was a matter of time now, just as Dr. Diamond had told me ten hours ago.

So I was to wait. Again.

After a while, I calmed down and recognized that things were not likely to change in the next few hours. Pam, Bruce and Karen had returned to the room and wondered if I needed anything, wanting to help me if they could. Despite their incredulous looks, I insisted we all go out and have a proper dinner. All of us needed to decompress, and I knew that in the ICU there would be little opportunity for us to engage in normal activity.

"Carolyn is going to be all right," I told them "and the ICU is the safest place for her. The nurses have my cell phone number if anything should happen." They silently accepted my wishes, and secretly concluded I was in deep denial. I could guess what they were thinking, "Surely he can see that she might die? Wouldn't he want to be here if that happened? We shouldn't leave her alone!" I led the way out of ICU and down the corridor, sure in my knowledge that Carolyn would be there when I returned.

Mark, who had been keeping the sleeping bags and stewed coffee company in the waiting room, joined the three managers and me. We invited Thomas to help again with the transport. The six of us left the hospital, but we didn't say a word about the day's drama, as if nothing had happened, and I was a visitor or guest, not a grieving spouse. After a few drinks at the dinner table, laughter and raucousness burst out of us. The levity and fun released the tension and rejuvenated our outlook. There were so many new faces to take in, although the discussion tended to revolve around me, as they were eager to hear about Australia. That was a safe, easy topic for all of us. I was becoming used to the attention and the fascination with my accent, having arrived in the country only a few months earlier. I even felt comfortable enough to point out that it was "them that had the accent, not moi"!

I was happy that the world had stopped spinning for a moment. I had woken in Boston, was served lunch somewhere over Missouri, and now I was having dinner in Texas with a bunch of strangers. The Mexican restaurant served as the perfect escape; richly colored with a jolly ambiance that held no hint of disaster.

❧

After dinner, I asked to be taken back to the hospital, so I could say good night to Carolyn. There had been no change, nothing to report. She looked peaceful enough, although not exactly healthy. I was pleased there had been no change. It was a good sign as far as I was concerned. If she stayed stable, she might just pull through. Sitting on the bed stroking her face, I noticed the blue polka dots on her gown matched both the blanket across her legs and the plastic cover on the pillow. Someone had braided her long blonde hair. I remembered that it looked freshly brushed when I had arrived a few hours earlier. I guessed that having her hair up helped keep it clean. Besides, it looked nice. She was obviously in good, caring hands. I said good night to the nurses, and headed off to another disturbing hurdle—her hotel room. It was sensible for me to occupy Carolyn's hotel room, as it was full of her things. It was, however, an emotional minefield, which I hadn't anticipated.

I opened the door, put my bag down and looked around. It was eerie and still, but slightly familiar. All hotel rooms look alike, even on the other side of the world! I couldn't help but look in the closet. I felt like an intruder, and slightly guilty at being there. The clothes hanging up had her scent, and I started to weep again. How could this be happening? Why did she have a cardiac arrest? What if it had happened here in this room? Who would have known?

Standing at the bathroom door, I noticed Carolyn hadn't had time to tidy up after the early morning rush. Her makeup bottles and lotions seemed scattered across the vanity, which surprised me, as she was so meticulous at home. I realized my influence didn't reach this far; she obviously let her hair down when alone, but it felt like I was catching her in a lie. I tidied them all up, and my teardrops sprinkled across the jars and tubes as I put them back into her makeup bag. I looked into the mirror, and told my reflection that maybe things were not going so well. I had to be brave, and face the harsh reality. Carolyn had had a traumatic episode and might not survive, no matter what I did or said.

I sat on the end of the bed, and looked at the TV. It looked back at me. My favorite CNN had no appeal, and I was not interested in flicking the channels, so that escape route was fruitless. The clipboard of hospital paperwork looked complicated. I could handle the easy parts: name, address and social security number. But the rest of it had to wait.

I was glad we had had the margaritas at dinner, and several glasses of wine, as I was in need of rest, and wanted the negative thoughts and fears to abate. Oh, please, stop the horror, and let me wake from this nightmare. Carolyn's nightie was under the pillow. I haven't needed a security blanket for many decades, but I clung to this one.

❧

The sun streaming in the window struck my face, waking me, and I opened my eyes to find myself in an unfamiliar room. Where am I? With the move from Australia, it had been several months since I had had a permanent bedroom, so I was not too disoriented. But I couldn't recall this room at all. I propped myself up on the pillows and looked out the window at the blazing sun, concrete driveway winding through grassy banks and stunted trees. Oh, I'm not in Salem or Melbourne. I'm in Dallas, in Carolyn's hotel room. I smiled at the realization that she had asked for an east-facing window. Every time we travel I ask for a room with morning sun, and she must have picked up my habit—there was no chance she could have known I would be sleeping in this room.

So that Friday morning I wouldn't be in our Salem apartment, honing my resume, searching the job banks, or telephoning potential contacts for informational interviews. I had been spending the time between our honeymoon and the green card interview getting a personal network established. My diary had been filling up quickly, and I was eager to get back into the corporate world after my few months "holiday" managing our "emigration". But all that was going to be in doubt now. The pessimistic thoughts took control again. What happens to my immigration application if she dies? Can I still stay here, or do I have to go back? What will I do without her? How quickly a bright future turns bleak. Our home in Australia was rented out, and our belongings were still on a container ship crossing the Pacific! I could not deal with all these complications. And they didn't even know what was wrong with her!

These thoughts, however, did make me eager to get back to the hospital. I knew it would be some time before I returned to the hotel, so I decided to make good use of the facilities. A clean-shaven face, fresh clothes and a full belly would help me conquer the challenges ahead. That was the plan, anyhow.

Down at the concierge desk I was treated like a VIP. I thought it was because of Carolyn's Hilton Honors membership status, but soon realized they knew why I was there—they were probably on duty when it happened.

"Good morning, Mr. Whitehead. How is your wife doing? We have a shuttle to take you to the hospital this morning, and please call me when you need to be picked up," said Keith, Director of Front Office Operations, as he handed me his business card. He then gestured towards the forecourt where I saw the ten-seat bus waiting. "How long will you need the room?" My eyes widened, my mouth dropped open, but no words emerged. He quickly continued, "I'm sorry. What I mean is, you can have the room as long as you need. I just want to give you enough breakfast vouchers." He then paused, "If there is anything we can do…"

I struggled to acknowledge the superb customer service and stammered my way through an answer. How on earth could I know how long I would be there? I guess they were as shocked as I was. Gold Card guests aren't supposed to collapse and die in their establishment, especially the employees of a major client.

Chapter 4

THREE DAYS TO LIFE

Our fear of death is like our fear that summer will be short,
but when we have had our swing of pleasure, our fill of fruit,
and our swelter of heat we say we have had our day.

–Ralph Waldo Emerson

My second day in ICU was a little easier. I had become used to the terminology and activities of the nurses, and they were getting to know me. They seemed to like having me around, and I built some rapport with the cheekier ones.

An intensive care unit is designed for observation and monitoring of life threatening illness. There is little distinction between night and day. Time is measured in terms of routines; administration of drugs, measurement and verification of life support equipment, fluids to go in, and fluids to be taken out. Unfortunately, this can cause severe psychological stress for the patients. The high noise level, unchanging light, lack of windows and clocks, combined with a clear view of other patients, can be disorienting, impair short-term memory (most likely due to the disturbed sleep pattern), and can also delay recovery. It even has a name—"ICU psychosis"!

Despite the rules to the contrary—which were prominently posted at the entrance—I was allowed to remain in Carolyn's room. It was really just a large glass fronted cubicle, with a floor to ceiling curtain. Apparently, I was a good influence, and encouraged to be there as her blood pressure and the all-important blood oxygen level improved whenever I was in the room. The peg on her finger was actually a pulse oximeter monitoring the oxygen saturation of her blood. Must keep it above ninety percent, I was told. That meant she had to breathe consistently and deeply. For nearly twenty hours she had had one hundred percent oxygen forced into her lungs because they were not working well enough. She had a reading of only seventy percent after the EMTs brought her in. With levels below eighty percent, the neurons do not receive enough oxygen to function normally, leading to unconsciousness. At thirty percent those cells are dying.

Periodically, the nurse would reduce the sedative to bring Carolyn out of sedation enough that they could assess her neurological condition. When they did this, Carolyn went into fits of thrashing about, but I was told this was normal behavior for someone who is intubated. Even though her frantic movement was a good sign, I found it disturbing. She was behaving like a mortally wounded animal, tied down and suffering the death throes. At least I could see she was alive. I asked about this magic trick they performed—making her suddenly animated.

When I touched her she calmed down so I spent a lot of time sitting on the side of the bed, stroking her face and holding her hands. During these "tests" we played a game, she would slowly lift her hand to grab the tube in her mouth, and I would guide it back down to the bed, sometimes resting it on my leg. I talked to her as though she was fully awake and perfectly healthy. I had no idea whether she could hear me or not, and anyway, I was probably doing it for my own wellbeing.

It was during these periods of her semi-consciousness that I gleaned some hope for the future. I wanted to find out more about the relationship between dosage and her level of consciousness. Maybe Carolyn would be able to communicate with me soon?

I also started to wonder about death, and what it would be like. Would Carolyn have known? And if she did, what would her last thoughts have been? Maybe she would have wanted to say, "Goodbye, I'll see you in heaven," as John D. Rockefeller Sr. purportedly said, on his deathbed, to Henry Ford. Or would she have been more like Charlotte Bronte and said to herself, "Oh, I am not going to die, am I? He will not separate us, we have been so happy." She could have been confused, and remarked, "Goodnight, my darlings, I'll see you tomorrow," as the playwright, Noel Coward said the night before he died in 1973. Would I ever find out what Carolyn thought? Would she ever be able to talk to me again? Not for the first time, I had to push the morbid thoughts away and concentrate on what I knew, not what I feared.

One of the nurses came in to give me a plastic bag with Carolyn's belongings, and to check a few administrative details with me. After the mundane paperwork details were confirmed, I was left alone to look inside the bag. Her shoes weighed the bag down, so I took them out. In the bottom of the bag was a scrap of cloth, torn and cut raggedly. I realized it was one of the blouses Carolyn had bought at the Kittery factory outlets, on the way back from our honeymoon in Maine. It was now ruined, but then I felt something underneath the destroyed piece of clothing. It was her watch, and still keeping time. The band was clasped around an invisible wrist, and threaded onto it were her wedding band and engagement ring. My eyes blurred, the tears welled up, and I started to sob again. They only give the personal effects to the next of kin, don't they? And usually after....

Maybe that's why they let so many of us into the ICU, because she wasn't expected to live. I refused to believe Carolyn was going to die. It wasn't possible. What on earth could be wrong with her that she was there at all?

࿚

Hospitals are full of people, and yet they can be the loneliest of places. I had never experienced so overpowering a sense of emptiness and isolation before, despite so many hours and days I spent alone as a child. I needed to leave that harsh, danger-filled ICU, and attempt to bring some normality back into my life. I decided that talking to people I knew could help. Although I had little new information, I felt I should relay the news on Carolyn's condition to her family. Also, I had not heard from her brother Dave, about his plans for coming to Dallas.

The hospital Chapel was at the end of the corridor, suspiciously close to the emergency room and ICU. I entered the sun filled room with its curved glass-brick walls, and sat on one of the benches. For me it was a quiet place, a refuge from the drama outside. The serenity in that space helped me relax. I gained a little strength from it, but decided to check my voicemail messages before talking to the family. I was feeling apprehensive, anticipating the raw emotions, both Helen's and mine, so I wanted to put off the call to her. However, Auntie Evie's voice interrupted my anxious thoughts. She had just heard the news and wanted to tell me they were praying for Carolyn. I had not spoken to her since the wedding, and welcomed the feeling of support from my new extended family. There was also a call from the hospital's administration, asking me to contact them about Carolyn's insurance details.

My call to Helen was full of tears and anguish and I naively thought the next call, the one to hospital admin, would be straightforward. I had no idea how complicated the American medical insurance game could be. Armed only with Carolyn's Blue Cross Blue Shield membership card, I entered a new world with its strange language and air of expectation that I knew what I was doing!

Luckily, I found sympathy in the hospital administrator's office. Carolyn's social security number plus the magic blue insurance card provided everything they needed—for the moment.

I was also told to contact my HMO and advise them of Carolyn's admission. The first hurdle I had to confront was trying to understand what an HMO was. Then, I had to work out how to get our Health Maintenance Organization bureaucracy to start serving me, rather than the other way around.

Within a minute or so into the call to Blue Cross, a new barrier was put before me. "Has your wife selected a PCP?" the curt customer service woman asked.

This was the very first decision point in the call and I realized I was going to need help. In Australia, PCP is what the crazy drug addicts take to get high, but I was sure that was not what she meant.

"I don't know. What is a PCP?" I replied.

"A Primary Care Physician, sir. You have to have a PCP to authorize any medical services."

"Maybe I should explain," I responded, thinking this was going to become a problem. "My wife has been admitted to the hospital with a sudden cardiac arrest. She is in intensive care and the hospital has asked me to advise you of her admission."

"Is this an emergency, sir?"

"Yes it is. She is in intensive care." Did she not listen to me the first time?

"Oh, you don't need a PCP for that," she answered, as if this is the most basic and obvious concept known to man. Well, not to this man!

What do I need one for then? I wondered. "How do we select a PCP?" I asked, in case someone said I *did* need one.

"Oh, I can give you the list. What zip code?"

I stumbled over my answer, since I was used to calling it a postcode, and she started to read out the names of doctors in our area, one after another as if they would mean something to me.

"I'm sorry but I don't know any of these doctors, I've only just arrived in the country. Can't we just select the first one on the list?" I asked.

"You have to ring them first to make an appointment, and they may not be accepting new patients."

I was close to exasperation. This reminded me of dealing with the government departments back home. Just as Yossarian had uncovered, in Joseph Heller's wonderful novel *Catch-22*, I was finding that every step you take has choices presented that require you to take the step, before you can determine what step you should be taking!

"Read out the addresses please, and I'll see if I can recognize any of the streets," I suggested.

Eventually, I selected a medical center not far from our apartment and got the contact details. Since I was feeling some prowess in handling the situation, I first confirmed with the HMO customer service agent my selection of our PCP. I could always change it if they weren't accepting new patients!

That accomplished the first part—a PCP had now officially been selected. Next, I had to find out if the PCP wanted to be selected! Yossarian would have been proud of my logic.

This next call was more of the same, but I was wise to the game now.

"I'd like to register as a new patient please," I asked the medical clinic receptionist as confidently as I could.

"When would you like to come in for the appointment?" she replied.

"I don't want to make an appointment, I want to register as a new patient." Was it my accent, or was I using the wrong words? Did she not understand me? How could I be so easily confounded by such a simple task?

Yes, sir, and when would you like to come in for your first appointment?"

"Maybe I should explain," I continued, thinking this was a déjà vu. "My wife has been admitted to the hospital with a sudden cardiac arrest. She is in intensive care, and the HMO has asked me to select a PCP.

"Is this an emergency, sir?"

"Yes it is. She's in intensive care!"

"Oh, you don't need an appointment for that," she answered. "All emergencies are automatically accepted by the health care provider, sir."

&

My brief sojourn outside the ICU, grappling with HMOs and PCPs was over, and I wanted to be with Carolyn again. Her appearance was so disheartening that I soon lost the glee of surviving the health insurance bureaucracies. Carolyn's arms looked like she had been beaten. Huge bruises covered both forearms, and her right arm was the worst—deep purple giving way to black and yellow. In addition, the skin on her face and arms was puffy and swollen. The bruises on her arms were so bad, that I asked one of my new friends what was causing them. The nurse replied with a very matter of fact tone, "When they 'stick you' in an emergency they don't have a great deal of time to be considerate."

"And what about the swelling?" I asked.

"She has been given a lot of fluids to keep her BP up, and it tends to make the arms and legs swell up. That's why we took her rings off." She looked at me directly and said, "You wouldn't have wanted us to cut those beautiful rings off, now would you?"

Certainly not!

I began to understand how much they cared. Their attention to detail was impressive. I recognized that she wanted me to appreciate how their actions were helping Carolyn, despite the appearances.

It was difficult to consider complaining about the consequences of Carolyn's emergency treatment, and it looked as though the EMTs had done the most damage. Maybe that's what the nurse wanted me to believe, so I would not feel so bad. Although, I did wonder about the fresh bruises, still growing mottled and red.

Not content with letting this damage continue, I asked the nurses what could be done to save Carolyn's arms; "surely there was a better way?" They seemed pleased with my question. They, too, wanted to avoid the trauma. I gathered there was some difficulty in finding the veins in Carolyn's forearms to start fresh IV lines. I was advised that patient's veins tend to close up with the powerful drugs being used and they needed to move the lines regularly, so it was likely to get much worse.

"We can put in a central line," I was told. That way all the IV drips would connect to a single tube, semi-permanently inserted into a large vein in Carolyn's chest. "It would be much better, as these drugs are very damaging to those fragile veins in her arms," the nurse continued.

Central venous catheters are usually performed under local anesthetic and intravenous sedation. The procedure is a relatively safe one, with few complications. I had no idea how long Carolyn was going to be in hospital, and her arms were taking such a beating. She was already sedated, so the procedure would be simple and quick. I was told to consider the short-term risks, such as an incorrect placement of the needle into the subclavian vein, which could puncture a lung, or cause bleeding into the chest; I acknowledged that these complications occur less than five-percent of the time.

The nurse looked at me with anticipation. I agreed to the central line. I could not bear to see them continue to use my wife as a pincushion—there were so many IV bags hanging up, and more were strung up every hour. Besides, the catheters in Carolyn's arms had to be changed so often, and those small veins in her forearms had less blood flow than the big one in her chest. I also wanted to avoid any potential damage from the medications irritating her delicate blood vessels. I could see the nurse felt it was the best choice.

Of course, this decision had ramifications. I was presented with a clipboard on which there were several forms requiring my signature. These consent forms were another first for me. First, the insurance mumbo-jumbo, and now this sudden exposure to the American medical indemnity world. I didn't exactly dread the legalese, but I wondered if I could be expected to understand the language, since my recent induction to HMOs and PCPs had hardly proven I was equipped for the job. It was curious that they could pump Carolyn full of powerful and dangerous drugs, and zap her many times with a defibrillator with impunity, but when it came to a procedure that would help prevent further damage, I had to take the responsibility!

I didn't hesitate, although I noticed the paragraphs of legal jargon providing the hospital with protection if there were any complications, most of which were duly pointed out by the doctor. I was reminded of Carolyn's habit of reading every line of any agreement before she signs. I had valiantly tried to point out that a telephone company or a bank was not likely to alter their contract for every customer, but it was always in vain. Carolyn felt she always had the option of not signing! In this case, what choice did I have?

It was not until much later that I found out what drugs Carolyn had been given, and their effects. One of them, the anti-coagulant heparin, was most likely causing the bruising to worsen. But that was just a shocking side effect, and not life threatening, so it was relegated to the bottom of the list of things to remedy.

I was not allowed to be present when they did the central line procedure. I was told to wait outside where there was a waiting room with coffee and TV. I did not follow this advice. I had mission to complete, and it was not to watch junk on TV. My more important task was to meet with Carolyn's saviors, Tom and Randy. They had been her artificial lungs and heart in the hotel conference room. I wanted to hear what actually had occurred, from their perspective. I hadn't been able to adequately answer the doctor's questions about what preceded her collapse, and I didn't trust the clinical hypotheses. I wanted to find out for myself. Exactly what happened, who did what, and how?

I was not sure what I might discover, but I had arranged with Mark for all of us to meet at the hotel. I wanted to thank both of them, as well as learning what had transpired the previous morning. Strangely, I felt I was intruding on these business people, reasoning that they only had two days for their course and that somehow it was my fault that the first day was ruined. In addition I was asking them to relive the harrowing experience. They could hardly say "no", and yet I felt uncomfortable. Mark introduced us and I shook their hands.

"Thank you for saving my wife. I have a few questions I need answered…" I blurted out.

Tom and Randy were clearly unsure what I sought. What could they say that wasn't already known?

"Maybe we should sit down?" Mark suggested.

Once we were settled and I had relaxed a little, I explained that the doctors had been asking me about the collapse—specific details such as: What were her facial expressions? How did she fall down? Did she say anything? Did she grab her chest?

Tom began, and as his words tumbled out, I jotted them down on the notebook I had instinctively brought from Boston.

The words looked terrifying, and I couldn't picture the event at all. They were just words I had written on the page. "Fell off chair sideways onto her face. Tremor. Labored breathing. Rolled her over, no response. Flushed red face. Breathing stopped. Nurse took over, pulse returned, face still blue. Faint sounds, eyes closed. Restarted CPR. Tongue movement. EMTs intubated her."

This was the first time I had heard any details about her collapse. I had a thousand questions of my own, but looking at the two of them I realized the questions could wait. I told them how grateful I was, and reiterated that I believed they had saved her.

Jim was watching me question Randy and Tom from the background and almost the minute I started talking, his earlier fears of my denial were dispelled. "Boy, this guy is quick to take charge and assume the responsibility. He is clearly a caring spouse, and the way he has gotten into the middle of it, he's as good a manager as I've seen," he wanted to say. "This guy is not the same person I spoke to on the phone yesterday." I was closer to my normal self at that point. I had a task to accomplish, and I was focused on the facts. But I was not the one to see her "lights go out" and so, understandably I had a different perspective.

I then asked if anyone knew where Kathy Williams, the nurse trainer who had helped with the CPR, might be, and if she was still in the hotel. Mark found her and brought her over to the group. She seemed apprehensive as I expressed my gratitude to her.

"Oh you don't need to do that, these boys did all the work," she said, gesturing towards Randy and Tom. She then asked about Carolyn's condition. I could see from Tom's expression that this was a difficult moment for him, and noticed that Randy had looked off into the distance.

"She is alive. She is in Intensive Care. They have her sedated and on a ventilator, but I want them to wake her up." Nobody said a word. I had to fill the void with words. I felt like a fool, "They don't know what is wrong with her, but it isn't an aneurism. Could have been a heart attack. Her ejection fraction is low. We have to wait for some more tests." Jim looked at his feet, Kathy smiled knowingly, but Tom and Randy just looked at each other and then down at the floor.

"Kathy, can I get your contact details…" I finally asked.

I had optimism. They had images of yesterday. I could not expect them to see my perspective, as much I could not accept theirs. I told them all again that, without them, Carolyn would not be alive. I thanked them for their courage and their willingness to act.

Everyone then dispersed, and I was left with my notes. Clearly my fact-finding mission was finished, but I just sat there. Mark gently reminded me that we had to get to the airport to pickup my brother-in-law. Dave had told me, in one of my earlier phone calls, that he had found a cheaper plane ticket, and would be arriving from Rhode Island around lunchtime.

I was now grateful to have someone to share the emotional burden. My earlier concerns about independence were replaced by a desire to have close company. Whereas I had innocently come to Dallas to bring my girl home, it was now obvious that we had to remain until the cause, and a solution, could be found. I had come to the realization that this was no minor ailment, and my preoccupation with Carolyn's tolerance to pain was both irreverent and irrelevant.

৽

My second visit to Dallas Fort Worth International airport was less remarkable than the first. I was understandably preoccupied with the story I had just heard, from the mouth that supplied Carolyn's breath and shaking the hands that had kept her blood flowing. We traveled in silence, taking the same road to the airport as last time, but this time in the opposite direction. I was worried about the pessimism I had perceived in Tom and Randy. What did they imagine that I hadn't been told?

I was also busy thinking about how to prepare Mark for the introductions. I didn't feel embarrassed, or intend to cast aspersions, but Dave's appearance is so at odds with his personality and demeanor. I decided to call it like it is.

"Mark, Dave looks fierce, but he is a really kind and gentle guy. He has a pony tail down his back, and will probably be wearing leathers." Mark just looked at me and nodded. "He works in drug rehabilitation for the state government." I continued, "He has great rapport with his clients." Mark nodded again and remained silent.

Waiting at the airport arrivals terminal, I decided not to worry about perceptions, and to just accept matters as they were—Que Sera Sera.

On my third tour of the baggage claim area, I was astounded to see someone I knew. I was expecting Dave, and he is not easy to miss, but I could not believe the sight in front of me.

"CJ! What are you doing here?" I said as I clapped my arm over his shoulder.

"Hi, Uncle Jeremy. I came to help Auntie Carolyn. She is very special to me," he replied with a smile, but also a worried expression.

CJ is the younger son of Carolyn's sister, Janet. He was in our bridal party, and I had enjoyed talking with him about his plans for the future. He was still in that wild eyed, wondrous age between teenager and adult.

Dave followed CJ out with the luggage, and I introduced them both to Mark. The surprise and excitement of seeing CJ was now replaced by a foreboding—Dave had asked how Carolyn was. I told him she was alive, but they didn't know what was wrong with her. I had little to offer in the way of details. Instead, I suggested we get them checked in at the hotel first, before going to see her. I was anticipating that we would stay at the hospital until late, and as Mark had already arranged the room for them, I wanted to inconvenience him as little as possible.

❧

Dave and CJ stood beside the hospital bed and just looked. They looked at me, back at Carolyn, and at the monitors. Then they looked at me again, and finally at Carolyn. Dave picked up her hand, but it stopped a few inches from the mattress.

"They have her tied down because she tried to pull the tubes out," I explained.

Dave nodded, and then spoke directly to Carolyn, "Carolyn. It's Dave, your brother. I'm here to help you. CJ is here too. We love you very much, and want you to get well." The tears trickled down his face, and his voice was low and halting.

Dave was preparing himself for Carolyn's death, thinking the only thing keeping her alive was the ventilator. He did not hold out much hope for her. She looked like death already. Dave had had some experience with death. The keyboard player from his rock'n'roll band had been placed on life support two years earlier, but did not survive. Two conflicting thoughts ran through his mind. "She's not going to make it. But, if she makes it through the night, she might come through okay."

CJ was clearly shocked by the sight of his favorite family member motionless and yet tied down, tubes and wires strewn across the bed covers, and her face seemingly composed by an embalmer. He said nothing, did nothing; he just stood there, his eyes locked onto Carolyn's face. His eyes brimmed with tears, they broke free and cascaded down his cheeks, but he made no sound at all.

≫

When Dave and CJ had recovered from the shock, and were relatively composed, I asked if they wanted anything; maybe the bathroom, or something to drink? They did not need to rebalance their bodily liquids. They did, however, need to revitalize their nicotine levels.

Mark suggested we might want a car to get about. He offered to get a rental car for me to use, but I deferred the decision to Dave, as I was comfortable with the hotel shuttle bus. I really only needed to go from my bed to Carolyn's, and back each day. Plus I was only just coping with driving around Massachusetts, (so unlike Australia, where we drive on the left hand side of the road), and didn't want the additional stress of negotiating with Texan roads and drivers.

Dave, on the other hand, couldn't see any sound reason not to have a car to drive around, so they headed off to get Mark's car from the parking lot.

"Want me to bring you back something to eat?" Dave asked on the way out.

In the few weeks I had been in America I had learned that this was a trick question, for you need to know what is available before you can answer! In Boston, I had a devil of a time finding something similar to what I would have for lunch back home. A sandwich here more often than not turns out to be a burger, or a roll with hot meat sauce, but in Australia, it is two pieces of multigrain crusty bread with several fillings like ham, cheese, tomato, and lettuce. And you don't get chips with it. The sandwich comes freshly made, wrapped in paper and is usually slipped inside a white paper bag. Not being a fan of McDonalds and the like, I was usually hard pressed to define anything my new countryman could order for me, and I certainly had no idea about those side options endlessly presented once that first decision had been made!

"No thanks, I'll get something from the cafeteria later," I said, deciding to avoid the whole concept of food selection. I wasn't so interested in changing the contents of my stomach anyhow—it was best to leave it alone. I had not yet learned the concept of comfort food.

✎

When the nurses weren't fiddling with the drug dosages or IV lines, Carolyn remained motionless, her chest moving up and down to the beat of the respirator, and the heart rhythm trace on the monitor continued endlessly, almost mesmerizing in its monotony. What little space there was in the room was taken up by the equipment, so I took up station on the edge of her bed. There was a chair, but it was specially designed for critically ill patients: the seat was close to the floor, and it had armrests that tilt back to allow side entry. I tried sleeping in it, the adjustable back and some rubber pillows made it slightly less uncomfortable than an airline seat. But sleep was no easier to achieve there, than in the sumptuous hotel bed. At that moment it felt like nothing was happening, and I had to remind myself that that was a good thing. Not much more than thirty hours ago there had been a lot of activity and none of it had been pleasant. That regular heartbeat I could see on the monitor, although now too fast, was non-existent then. Those breaths I could hear had not been there, not to mention the fact that she had had no blood pressure at all. So things were a lot better now. But why did this occur? What could be wrong? Was Carolyn really going to survive? Shouldn't we be doing something to cure her? What good was there in waiting?

Studying the monitor became a new occupation of mine. What were all those numbers and letters for? What could they tell me? I recalled the nurse's explanation. There were four critical things being measured: her heart rate, her blood pressure, the blood oxygen level, and her respiration rate. The top squiggly line was yellow and showed her heartbeat in real time. The number next to it was her heart rate and it was hovering around one hundred twenty-five. But she was lying absolutely still, and that's how fast her heart used to pump when she was pounding up the hill on our walks! The next set of numbers showed her blood pressure, and those green digits did not look healthy at all, ninety and sixty-five. One is the systolic the other is the diastolic, I couldn't remember which was which, but I knew that "ninety over sixty-five" was too low. A healthy reading would be something like one-twenty over eighty. So her heart was banging away furiously, and yet not able to provide a healthy pressure.

Watching those nurses work tirelessly and patiently, it soon became apparent to me that they are the real caregivers. They were soothing and empathetic, patient and careful in their explanations. I consider nurses to have the most difficult job, since they can't hide behind a mask and escape into terminology to conceal what is going on. Hardly an hour went by without Carolyn undergoing some form of clinical procedure, and yet the nurses treated her as a sensitive and needy human being who was scared and confused. Even though she showed no signs of being able to appreciate it—she could not see, could not hear and could not talk—yet they cared for her as though she was awake and alert.

The day wore on with little or no indication of time passing. Dave had returned from getting the rental car, so I decided to take a break. The waiting was unrelenting. Inactivity is not my specialty and I thought that stretching my legs with a walk around the hospital corridors could help distract me. I stopped by the cafeteria to see what I had missed out on, and then I did a cursory check of the captives in the waiting room, all the while wishing for a miracle.

I needed those little escapes from the ICU, to counter the image before me of Carolyn motionless with her life force preserved only by the machines. Most of the time I felt like a zombie, and at best like flotsam and jetsam floating on the wind or water, being pushed here and there. I was unsure of my role, and whether there was anything I could do to have my beautiful bride back.

❧

Finally, it was time for the evening rounds and Dr. Hecht arrived a little breathless, holding the ubiquitous clipboard chart. He looked tired, as he ran his eyes down the pages, "Well her BP is stable, although a little low, she is sinus tachycardia. Sorry, her heart is beating too fast, with some abnormal rhythms. Her blood chemistry is also abnormal, possibly from alcohol abuse?" He gave me that intense penetrating stare again, as though he was a psychiatrist or an alcoholic's counselor, and expecting me to lie. He quickly looked down again and continued in that harried voice, "The neurological exam is inconclusive; she needs more time for us to get a better indication. I suspect she has a malignant ventricular arrhythmia with occult coronary artery disease." He looked up again, and seeing my blank expression added, "she has blockages in her arteries that has damaged the heart muscle and is causing the abnormal rhythms."

While I was following him better than the previous day, the story hadn't changed much. He was postulating that her heart was damaged from blocked arteries. But I wanted more than guesses. "Tell me exactly what is wrong and what needs to be done, and tell me soon. This uncertainty is unbearable." I did not let these thoughts escape into my mouth, but I am sure they were written all over my face.

"So how long until we know if she is…. When can she be taken off the sedation?" I didn't really want to hear any more bad news, and until she was awake I couldn't make my own assessment!

"Well, the pulmonologist would need to make that decision. I recommend an angiogram to locate the blockages. I'll look at scheduling it for early next week," he said, followed by another one of his piercing looks. "We'll see how she progresses over the next few days." Dr. Hecht looked at me expectantly, so I nodded and gazed over towards the bed. I was just a spectator, and neither ready nor qualified to make a judgment. He was the expert, I would defer to his advice. After making a few notations he left, with a short aside, "I'll talk to Dr. Siminski, the pulmonologist. Good night."

CJ was seated on the chair, busy doodling with pen and paper, while Dave was standing vigil over the bed. Neither had said much and I guessed they, too, were wondering what the outcome was going to be for Carolyn. I could not help but feel uncertain. Never before had I seen so many experts consulted and none offer a definitive answer. It was incongruous with my engineering mindset.

The despondent mood reminded me of the previous night, with Carolyn's managers, and I decided to treat Dave and CJ to dinner in the hotel restaurant. I needed a stiff drink, and they needed to adjust to the situation, so I chose a setting of calm and splendor. We sat at a table by the courtyard, away from all the other guests. Neither of them were drinkers. Dave had seen too much alcohol abuse and CJ was too young, so I was going to be drinking alone. The waiter brought over a martini, a glass of milk and a non-alcoholic beer. We had an uncertain time ahead of us and I sought to share some conventional activity that might help ground us. The last time we had all been together was the wedding reception, so a fancy dinner was fitting. I knew they would appreciate it, and told them to order whatever they wanted, and not to worry about the cost—I certainly wasn't concerned.

The courtesy newspaper was still at my hotel room doorstep when I retired and I noticed that the stock market had gained over three percent that day. At least Wall Street saw a rosy future.

~

When I awoke on October 12th, 2002, it was not a typical Saturday morning. Carolyn was not snuggling up beside me, and there was no reading in bed until late. But I knew where I was and why I was there. No surprises this time. It would have been nice to pull the blanket over my head and shut out the reality. Instead, I had to contain my excitement over breakfast with Dave and CJ. There was a chance Carolyn would wake up today, and then I would see if my little girl was the same or not.

From the moment the doctors had told me that Carolyn was deliberately paralyzed, I wanted to have her taken off the sedation. I understood their reasons and didn't object to them, I just wanted to have Carolyn awake and talking to me. Over the years I had seen how she would fight, most often railing against adversity and mediocrity in the workplace, and I would not accept the implication that she had a weak heart. My darling wife was strong and determined. She was not in any way ready to die. Surely that was obvious to them all. I had seen that she was breathing on her own and didn't need the respirator. There were at least four or five extra breaths displayed on the monitor than those set on the ventilator. This, too, should be obvious to the medical staff. Did they not see?

As soon as we arrived at the ICU ward I saw there had been no change to her condition, no improvement, but no deterioration either. It was further evidence to me that Carolyn was not going to leave me; she was not ready. So I asked the nurse to explain the process of bringing Carolyn into the conscious world.

"It is a simple matter of reducing the amount of sedative until she reaches that twilight zone, just like waking up from a deep afternoon nap," she told me.

I was eager to see something more than this lifeless shell with only a monitor on the wall to tell me she was alive. I wanted to see Carolyn open her eyes and look at me. I wanted to see her smile and watch her eyes light up as I had every morning when she awoke at home.

"This blue machine, called an infusion or volumetric pump," the nurse continued, "regulates the drugs she is being given. The dosage levels are displayed here." She pointed to the bright green LEDs. The section controlling Carolyn's sedative was set to forty-two. What an incredible coincidence—I had just turned forty-two years old, and we had been married on my birthday. It was also "the answer to the meaning of life" according to the *Hitchhiker's Guide to the Galaxy*. Many times I used this number to answer mundane questions for which I didn't have an answer, such as; "What is the temperature going to be today?"

So when can we wake the sleeping princess? Why not now! I wanted to demand, but I silently accepted the news that all it would take was an adjustment to the infusion pump and Carolyn would be back with me again. At least I had something concrete to grasp, some hard data to work with; adjust the dial and she would awaken. We were making progress, but my positive outlook did not create a glow on Dave's face, and CJ was preoccupied with his doodling. Did they know better?

Resigned to waiting again, I was surprised when, without any fanfare or hoopla, the nurse entered the room and began to reduce the dosage setting on the sedative. She looked at me and smiled but didn't say a word. Gradually the LED readout digits counted down. When the LED reached twenty-five Carolyn started to move about. I wanted it to read zero because then she would be alive again. I wanted to take her home; she didn't belong there. I was sure that once she was awake they would see that nothing was wrong with her.

Within a few minutes we would know what state her mind was in.

I was excited and apprehensive. I wanted that breathing tube out so she could talk to me, however I didn't want to know that she was mentally incapacitated—a vegetable. She could not stay like that, pipes and tubes forever.

Suddenly, Carolyn groaned and began to thrash about; her head shook from side to side, and her legs kicked the blankets off. Her arms struggled against the restraints, her fingers clenched into a fist and then extended fully out. I could see the tendons in her hands straining, making them look like chicken's feet. A moan escaped past the tube in her mouth. But her eyes stayed shut.

"Carol. Carol you are in hospital," the nurse yelled. She bent down and took Carolyn's hand in hers. "Carol can you squeeze my hand? Carol look at me. Carol."

I interrupted to explain that my wife's name was Carolyn. Not that it mattered much. Carolyn's sister Janet calls her Carol whenever they speak on the phone—never in person, just on the phone. Whenever she called Janet, long distance from Australia, I'd put my ear to the handset to hear the strange accents and different inflections.

I'm not sure why this sprang to mind, but it was not an ordinary time. This was the moment we would see if Carolyn was okay. Or not. She had been heavily sedated for two days; paralyzed to help her heart mend itself. But what about her brain?

The LED hit twenty and her eyelids snapped open. Her eyes looked murky and vacant. Oh, no! My heart stopped, and my stomach dropped. She appeared autistic, or very, very drunk. I started weeping, whether from shock and fear that she was brain damaged, or just overwhelmed that she was alive; no longer a lifeless mannequin lying on the bed.

I started babbling, "Darling you're all right. Oh my gorgeous little girl. You are in hospital. I love you very much. Do you understand?"

Incredibly, she turned to face me. I saw her eyes attempting to focus and a tear trickle down her cheek. I saw the pleading look pass across her face as the nurse began yelling again, "Carolyn, squeeze my hand."

She did. "You are in Baylor Hospital intensive care unit. You have a problem with your heart. You have a tube in your throat to help you breathe." Carolyn turned away from me, towards the nurse. The nurse stood up straight and seemed to relax a little. I watched her face for a sign. Her professional assessment appeared to be positive, but she said nothing. We couldn't be having false hopes. Or maybe it was a demarcation issue; only the doctors should diagnose?

It was clear that Carolyn could not comprehend what the nurse had just said. But it did register, and she wasn't panicking, which gave us all hope. She closed her eyes and her face relaxed, but then immediately she opened them again and blinked several times quickly. She appeared a little deranged and confused. Carolyn was alive, but she did not look normal. Her behavior was odd.

Dave and CJ were talking to her, I was cooing, and the nurse backed off to let us get closer to the bed. I could see that Carolyn was very confused, and yet there was a glimmer of hope; she seemed to recognize what was going on around her. Her eyes followed our voices. She tried swallowing, and then grimaced in pain. Her arm slowly lifted off the bed, her hand was attempting to claw at her face but the restraints did not let it get close enough and her arm fell back to the bed. She tossed her head back and forth, and a big frown creased her smooth forehead. I looked up to the nurse, my face silently pleading, "What can we do to ease the distress?" I was aware of the apparent contradiction in my wishes; they had sedated Carolyn to reduce the suffering!

But the nurse's expression was calm and relaxed; she almost seemed pleased. I realized that Carolyn had passed the test. Looking directly into Carolyn's eyes, the nurse said, "I'm going to lift you up a bit, so you can see a little better. But you can't pull the tube out of your mouth." It was a command, not a suggestion.

Carolyn accepted the statement and let her head fall back to the pillow, but now she could look around the room, not straight up into the bright ceiling lights. After several minutes of consternation Carolyn realized that she could not talk, and became agitated. She had a wild look about her, one I had not seen before and my heart sank again. But then, I realized she could feel the tube in her throat and didn't understand that it was there for a very important reason.

Carolyn had no energy and was able to keep her eyes open for no more than a minute at a time. But each time she opened them she looked as though she wanted to tell me something.

After about thirty minutes of anguish, I sought to pacify her and suggested she try to communicate by using my writing pad and pen. Carolyn had barely enough energy to hold the pen upright, let alone actually make a mark on the page.

"It's all right darling, we can talk later. I love you." She looked at me as though I was an imbecile, and tried again. This time she managed a vertical line that ended in a jagged tail. She was desperate to tell me something, and I wanted to appease her.

The hieroglyphic looked somewhat like the letter "h". I made a conspicuous guess, "It hurts?" Instantly, her eyes widened, her eyebrows shot up, and she moved her head towards me a fraction. It was as close to a nod as she was capable. She had exhausted herself with this momentous task and falling back on the pillow she closed her eyes.

I stroked her head and told her that she was going to be all right. "You had a cardiac arrest and they have put a tube down your throat to help you breathe." Her eyes opened again. "I know it hurts, it will be taken out soon." I told her this in the hope that it would comfort her, as she looked so distressed. Again she tried swallowing, scrunching up her forehead and jutting out her chin. I watched her hands like a hawk in case she tried to grab the tube. While it did feel cruel to have her awake and enduring the discomfort, I was being selfish and reveling in the elation that she was awake and alive. And she seemed able to easily comprehend our words.

Carolyn wanted to write something again, even though it was exhausting to merely lift a hand, and she couldn't co-ordinate her fingers so the pen would continually fall to floor. I held the pad, and put the pen in her hand, wondering if she knew that handwriting was almost impossible to achieve in her state.

The will was there but the strength was missing, and she produced abstract artwork instead of words. Carolyn could not accept that her fingers were not obeying; the pen did not stay upright in her hand and her arm slid down the page leaving a squiggly line, very similar to the blue and green traces on the heart monitor above her bed.

Her frustration with being unable to communicate was building, and she made a determined effort to write again. Now we had the perplexing game of guessing the first character she was attempting to write, and what the word might be. Dave and CJ felt compelled to assist, as they could not bear to see her so frantic.

Just as she was getting the second letter started, her arm lost the battle with gravity, and the pen scratched across the page. It was almost comical, or probably more like a toddler on the first attempt. We sat back and waited for her to recover.

Carolyn finally gained the strength to write one word, but none of us could decipher it! Were those first three letters "hun"? Was that a "y" at the end? There was a "u" and an "r" also and every attempt had begun with a vertical, sometimes two verticals like a capital H.

"What about 'hurts'?" I ventured.

She looked up and managed to nod once. We had already established this point earlier, but I acknowledged her desperate need to communicate, and started to ask questions in the hope I could guess what it was she wanted to tell us. I asked her to tap the pad once with her finger for yes, and twice for no. Tapping seemed a better idea than blinking for yes/no answers; after all she was closing her eyes more often than she blinked anyway!

"Your throat hurts?" I started with the easiest question.

Carolyn turned her head from side to side very slowly, any slower and it could have been misconstrued. She was shaking her head, NO. This was confusing, as we had already determined that her throat did hurt, just a few minutes earlier. She lifted her arm and her hand started the journey to her face again. "No, you can't pull the tube out," I said too quickly.

She gave me a fierce look and bent her fingers towards her chest. I hadn't meant to admonish her, but we were taking a liberty with the nurse's clemency in having the restraints loosened enough for Carolyn to hold the pen and write. Carolyn is an assertive, resolute woman who is often passionate in matters of control. She likes to be in charge of her world and can be difficult to reason with when she perceives things are not going her way. She looked at me in that familiar way—don't tell me what to do! I was pleased to see this trait reappear. It is not often that one is pleased with a spouse's ornery habits, but in this case I was overjoyed.

Was that a signal—touching her chest in that particular way?

"Oh! Your chest hurts."

She tapped the pad once.

I said, "You were given CPR at the hotel and they probably pushed too hard, so your ribs will be sore." I had hoped this explanation would end the discourse, or at least satisfy her need to communicate her pain, but she started with the pen again.

It was easier this time to guess the words she was trying to write. Finally she succeeded. She had exhausted herself to inform us that there was a tube down her throat! Also, that she had difficulty breathing, her chest was sore, and the tube was making her gag. These messages were not news to any of us. All of us had told her those precise details several times, in addition to those unambiguous commands from the nurses.

I became worried that Carolyn was not remembering things. I did not want to consider that prospect at all. As a diversion, I started to explain that she had to pass a breathing test before they would remove the tube. That got her attention and she lay back to listen to me.

"Your breathing was assisted by this ventilator." She slowly looked over at the machine I was pointing to, next to the bed. "It is not helping you now and that's why it is hard to breathe." I paused, and then continued in a serious tone, "You need to breathe deeply and regularly to show them you can breathe by yourself. Then they will take the tube out." I hoped she would not sense my desperation, although I am sure it was plainly evident. She needed to try hard, to overcome the pain and difficulty. But, did I want her to do it for me, or for herself?

As I had been told several times by the nurses, the most important criteria was Carolyn's blood oxygen level, called pulse-ox. She had to maintain better than ninety percent, without assistance from the ventilator, and breathing just room air. When she arrived in ICU, they had her connected to a respirator with one hundred percent oxygen forced into her lungs; six hundred milliliters, twelve times per minute. Yesterday, they had reduced it to only forty percent oxygen. Now the ventilator was switched off, and she was struggling a little on the room air, which was only around twenty percent oxygen. But the magic number stayed above ninety. I was so proud of my "fighter".

Throughout the morning, Carolyn wasn't able to do much more than lie still and stare at us, but she often gave a big slow sigh, probably from the exertion of breathing through the machine, rather than impatience. It reminded me of the exasperated sigh that my golden retriever, Waldo, used to give when he felt he had waited long enough to go for a walk. Most often I would be busy at my desk, or I'd be reading a book with him at my feet, and he would take a big breath and a long sigh followed by a miniscule shift of his head, bringing those sad eyes to bear on my face. It hardly ever worked, but I loved the cute look on his face all the same; those eyebrows wrinkled and arched just so. Now it looked as if my wife had learned the same trick!

We had to wait for the pulmonologist to give the all clear, but I was feeling very confident Carolyn would pass the breathing exam. I assured her the tube would be removed shortly. She became submissive in anticipation, silently looking into my eyes, trusting my words. We held hands as I sat beside her on the bed. She was so patient, enduring those long hours with a tube eight inches long and as thick as my finger stuck in her mouth, passing over her tongue, pushing past the epiglottis and down through her vocal chords. I could not imagine how uncomfortable it was.

Finally the moment we had been waiting for arrived. The pulmonologist walked in and asked the nurse how Carolyn had performed. I realized the test had actually been underway during the last few hours! So now it took only a confirmation by the nurses to the doctor and the extubation order was signed.

We were asked to leave the room while they removed the life support tool. I guess it was not going to be a pleasant sight, and besides, there was not enough room in the cubicle for all of us.

❧

Carolyn had a complete memory blank—nothing before, and not much after. She knew who we were, and that was certainly good news. She could now sit up in bed and move her head around unimpeded. She remembered that Dave was there, but got a surprise to see CJ. The tears welled up in her eyes, and tumbled down her cheeks. Her mouth distorted but no sounds emerged. I took her in my arms and held her tightly. I could feel her sobs; they were not much more than little hiccups since her chest and throat were so painful. I kissed her full on the mouth knowing that she would resist me and enjoy it in unison. But I was a little too greedy and she turned her head away. Carolyn coughed as though she was choking, and immediately put her hands to her chest and winced. "Oh, to be free of the tube, but how it hurts," she could not say. She smiled at me and wagged her finger—I had to be careful, and my excitement had overruled my sensibilities. Dave and CJ were next to hold Carolyn, but were so afraid to touch her that they executed the perfect air kiss and Hollywood hug. If she had been made of whipped cream, they wouldn't have marred the surface.

We had so much to talk about, but Carolyn had no energy, and no voice either. Being intubated for three days had irritated her vocal chords and throat, making speech painful and almost inaudible.

Her relief came in the form of ice chips, a simple and easy remedy but one that elicited an odd response. Carolyn looked in horror at the cup overflowing with crushed ice and clamped her mouth shut. I could see the words as though I was an expert lip reader, "my teeth are sensitive, don't put too much in my mouth!" Using a plastic spoon, Dave slipped one tiny piece of ice past her lips and we watched her face light up with delight. Up till now Carolyn had had all her fluids fed intravenously and her mouth was furry and dry. The sweet sensation of cool melting ice trickling down her throat transformed her. She almost glowed—almost.

A few more spoonfuls and the tears began again. We soon learned to accept her spontaneous crying; it seemed to be a constant release mechanism. I, too, became overwhelmed on a regular basis, and also had to let the emotions flow. Carolyn was awake and alive. But why did this happen at all? What was wrong with her? When will they be able to tell us? Could she give us any clues?

Several hours later, Carolyn started murmuring some exploratory words. Her voice was husky and dry, but recognizable. She was uncomfortable lying in the bed, and wanted to get out! After consultation with the nurses, we helped Carolyn expand her territory, and in the process we found out where that pink rubber tube went! There was a bag of yellow fluid attached to it that I recognized as one the nurses frequently checked and removed to measure the contents. That pink tube was just another reminder that there is no personal space in a hospital, no secrets and no privacy of bodily functions.

Helping Carolyn to sit in the chair was a superhuman effort. First she had to slide off the bed, and then she could toddle over using the IV stand as a crutch. After collapsing into the chair she wriggled about and we rearranged all the tubes, wires and bags. Finally she was settled and you could see the relief in her face—the pressure on her legs and back had changed. She had started the process of feeling normal, not bed ridden. The effort, however, had exhausted her, and she took a nap right there and then in front of our eyes. No warning, just "lights out". When she awoke it was a new day. Well it was for her. To us it had just been a twenty-minute interlude.

Each awakening was followed by three questions. Where am I? What day is it? What happened? And so it went, asking again and again and again. I became frustrated and sick of these same questions over and over. I was not resentful, but it was draining after a while. I decided to write the answers on the whiteboard conveniently mounted on the wall near the window of bricks. When Carolyn next asked the trio of questions I just pointed to it and asked her, "What does it say?"

On the first line, I had written in large green letters the current day and date. Next we had the name of the hospital. Then in larger letters were the words "Cardiac Arrest", and the date and time it happened. All I had to do was to get Carolyn used to looking up at the board when she woke up and wanted to ask.

Dave watched the two of us acting out this ritual in silence. In less than an hour Carolyn and I had been through the cycle half a dozen times: She would ask, "Where am I?" I would point to the board; she would ask, "What day is it?" I would remain silent and point to the board again. Finally, she would ask, "I had a cardiac arrest?" Then the tears began anew, each and every time.

Dave asked me why I was doing this. I told him it was for my own survival. I had already answered these interminable three questions fifty times already! I did feel a bit guilty, and hoped he was not going to tell me off. He surprised me. Instead of scolding me, he said that he was impressed. He told me that it was a technique he had seen used for people with brain damage and amnesia. He said the process allows the patient to connect the answers to a physical location, which assists them in rebuilding memories, and reduces the distress of not being able to remember details. He wanted to see if I knew that, and whether I was using it as a method to help Carolyn. To me, it was pure selfishness. I was tired of answering the same questions every time she woke up thinking it was a new day and not knowing anything!

ও

Jim usually doesn't answer his cell phone when at home, so it was strange that he answered my call that particular Saturday afternoon.

"Jim, this is Jeremy. She is awake. They took the breathing tube out this afternoon." I decided not to continue, as I did not want him to know about the memory problems just yet.

"That's the best news I've ever heard," he replied, "It's like being given a hundred Christmases at once."

I quickly realized that was the perfect comment to end the call, and I felt pleased that Jim had some good news for the weekend. He had not had such a good ending to the week, and could probably do with a boost. I also sensed that he was very surprised. It was not the outcome he was expecting at all.

This time, Jim was the one in disbelief over what he had heard coming out of the telephone handset, "How is it possible? I saw her lying there. I saw the lights go out," he said to himself after hanging up the phone.

～

Returning from my call to Jim I noticed the lack of food service in an ICU. The patients are not in a position to eat, and the nurses are too busy. So, no hospital meals in this ward, and maybe that was a good thing. No bathrooms either! Even more strange, was the absence of smells—I was only aware of sights and sounds— smell and taste were unnecessary senses in there. The fluorescent lights were on all day, all night, and every day of the week. In that ward the term twenty-four by seven has real meaning, and there was little sense of time, although you could use the routine of the nurse's supervision to get some indication if it was morning, evening or night. So it was not surprising that Carolyn was confused, each time she woke up could well have been a new day; nothing in the ICU would have contradicted it!

I have not watched a baby grow and develop, or a toddler learn to talk and walk. But watching Carolyn come out of her fug, dealing with the confusion about where she was, what happened and why, was how I imagined an infant would behave. She would look around the room and endeavor to decipher the meaning of her existence there. She would look towards the whiteboard and recall the reason for her hospitalization, but it was obvious she did not perceive the significance of being in an ICU. I suspect she was unable to assimilate any more than the fact that she had suffered a cardiac arrest and survived. Would that change? She was able to read and write, surely she could think as well?

Sleep seemed to be a natural therapy, as Carolyn could not remain awake for more than twenty minutes or so. There was one reward to this and I exploited it voraciously. Every time she woke, it was a new day for her, and she did not remember that I had brought some of her personal items from home. Thus, I was able to tell her about these "presents" many times over. Usually after she recovered from her bewilderment that the answers to her trio of questions were already written on the whiteboard, I would announce, "Darling, I have some presents for you!"

Then I would take out the overnight bag and hold out her comfy clothes, which brought a smile to her face. At least she remembered that part. Next would come her slippers, as I watched the smile become a tiny laugh. Then I would finish off with the coup-de-grace— her toothbrush. That's when I got the real reward, a big hug and a kiss for being so thoughtful.

CJ was jealous of this trick, "I can't believe the mileage you're getting out of this!" he said in a whisper, "That must be the tenth kiss you've got for the one present."

The toothbrush was especially cherished but the nurses advised that until Carolyn could swallow, she had to wait. I had brought some toothpaste as well, and a Styrofoam cup of water. I put them on the windowsill, next to the angels.

❧

Sunday was a special day. Carolyn was no longer sedated, and hopefully able to talk. I was eager to get over to the hospital, but I was not yet confident enough to drive in the unfamiliar town on my own, and of course I couldn't leave without my nephew and brother-in-law. I knocked on their door to give them a hurry-up. CJ was still not dressed, but Dave was ready to go. We told CJ to meet us down at the dining room. By the time we had finished breakfast, there was still no sign of CJ. Dave went to feed his nicotine habit, and I started off down the corridor to find my errant nephew. I tried to curb my impatience, telling myself that we would have all day to talk to Carolyn, so there was really no need to rush.

Eventually, we got to the hospital, after Dave pointed out the route so I could drive myself there and back. He was subtly getting me to realize that they would not be able to stay forever; he and CJ had to go back to their jobs and reassure our family in person.

As we entered the ICU, the nurses hurried over, their bright happy faces welcoming me back. I got the impression they were excited to listen to my accent again, but they were actually pleased to have me back in the ward because Carolyn was asking for me. When I entered, her eyes sparkled and she reached out her arms, with her fingers wiggling like a child does. Carolyn was hardly able to talk, although she looked somewhat normal, sitting up in bed beaming at me. She was still confused about her circumstance, understanding what had happened as though it had occurred to someone else. Denial is a powerful tool and sometimes operates in strange ways. It was not the time for me to correct her perception; we still had no idea of what was wrong with her heart, and so a little denial would be useful.

Carolyn was eager to show me a short note she had written for me that Sunday morning, showing her new perspective of the world.

"It's days like these that remind one to feel appreciative of every day that one feels well, except of course for the days when one has a hangover."

And she signed it with both her old initials *"CAB"* and the new ones *"CAW"*. There couldn't be too much wrong with her mind then! I looked over at Dave and I saw that he, too, was pleased with this sign of her intelligence.

&

"Were there angels watching over me?" Carolyn suddenly croaked, "Dave told me that I saw the angels." I wondered how long she had been mulling over this fact. We had been sitting silently for over an hour while Dave and CJ replenished their nicotine levels, and called home with updates on her condition. Carolyn had to know if it was true, since she was having great difficulty trusting her memory. Maybe it was a dream, or had angels really visited her when she was clinically dead?

"Yes, that's what you said, darling," I replied and then pointed at the window sill, "look, there they are!" She looked back at me confused, and looked at the window again. Her eyes twinkled once she realized that I was pointing at the figurines that Pam and Karen had bought the day she was admitted.

"You are so naughty! But I dreamed of angels. They were watching over me." She paused, "Is that why I'm still alive?" Tears burst forth, and the pain from the sobs pierced her chest like a scalpel. She cried out in agony, her ribs and chest were so painful, even more so now that she had been exercising them with all the talking and moving about. I stroked her back gently, and offered calming words. I had no clue how long the anguish was going to last, and did not know how to help. Is there anything that can take away the pain of despair?

Looking into her eyes, I could see we both struggled with the same dilemma. Was it better for her to forget? It would be so easy to let the past slip away in the night—pretend that she had not really been in danger. Or was this episode in our new lives so profound that we needed to face it directly; to understand intimately what had occurred and why; to look for reasons and remedies; to alter our outlook and plans for the future. How could we possibly live with the specter of sudden cardiac death striking again?

৯

Later that afternoon, it became obvious that Carolyn was no longer in a critical condition. She could breathe on her own, had a regular heartbeat and could talk, although only in short spurts. Dave and CJ had decided to make the most of their time and see some of the sights Dallas had to offer. They sheepishly asked me if that was okay, and wondered if I might want to come along. I gave Carolyn the choice and she thought it was a good idea. In her mind I needed to get to know my brother-in-law, and she thought this excursion could help him see the wonderful person she had married. She was worried, however, about what time we would be back. She had only just begun to comprehend how sick she was and didn't want to be alone for too long. I assured her we would not be long, and contemplated that she would probably sleep most of the time anyway. In addition, she was still not able to discern the passage of time very well. An hour to her was like five minutes, and so the hours slipped by quickly.

Relieved that Dallas had not taken my special person away, I was now quite interested in seeing a tribute to the country's youngest president—youngest to be elected *and* youngest to die. I stood on that spot painted on the road where the bullets hit his motorcade, and reflected that JFK was not much older than me at the time. He was in Dallas on business, politics of course, which led to his death. Carolyn was also there on business, but she had only clinically died. And the politics of her business were not extraordinary.

For me, and probably most of the population, Dealey Plaza was a scene from TV biographies, not a major road with fast moving traffic. And the grassy knoll was a blurry black and white photo or video image, not a park at the end of Main Street. It felt unreal to be standing in the Texas School Book Depository, looking through the suspect window, and seeing the forensic analysis of where the bullets went and what effect they had. I had enough horrors of my own to think about and sought solace in the gallery of Pulitzer Prize-winning photographs. Some of them depicted tragedies, but many of the scenes were peaceful, capturing the beauty of the world and its people in an instant, holding time quite still. I was unsure whether I wanted time to stand still, or quickly rush past this nightmare.

When we returned to Carolyn's bedside, her face was very pale and she looked scared. I had a terrible feeling that something was wrong, was she having a relapse? I looked up to the monitor to see if her vitals were in good shape. The numbers and wiggly lines were as they should be, so what could be wrong?

Reassured that her vital organs were functioning properly, I looked for some other cause. There was an eerie familiarity to her expression. Carolyn was behaving like Waldo again, this time fretting that she had been abandoned, but also relieved that we were back. Carolyn had never met Waldo, the golden retriever of my childhood. In fact, his name was chosen before mine, and from the same baby-naming book! It is such a magnificent name that my parents used it for each new dog, and as they all had identical traits, there was no more fitting a name. But now, Carolyn's expression and husky voice were perfectly imitating him. Waldo had once run away—escaped really—and was picked up by the dogcatcher to spend the night at the dog pound. When I retrieved him, he was hoarse from barking all night. He also looked frightened and yet was so excited to see me—exactly the same expression as Carolyn had on her face as we walked into the ICU. She was distraught that we had left and not said goodbye. But we had. She had no recollection of that, although she knew we had been there earlier.

We all talked at length about the possibility of us leaving the room and her forgetting we would be coming back. She agreed to write a note to herself that would help her remember the next time, such as when we went for dinner.

Carolyn showed just how smart she is by writing the note as a letter to us, written before we left. She even included some trick words to help her recall writing the note.

"*Thank you for coming to see me in eye see you.*

I know you will come back after dinner and that we said goodbye. But I still feel a little weird.

I love you."

I kept those scraps of paper with her notes and questions on them to look at again in the hotel room. They were so tender, and I pictured her sitting up in bed scribbling away. She insisted I read all of her notes, as her throat was raw and her voice was not much more than a whispered squeak. The next one was more poignant.

"He told me I said I dreamed of angels. You may have told me that but I didn't remember."

And another was a little disturbing.

"Do I have heart disease? I'm only 47 could it be Ginko Biloba?"

I had discussed with the ER doctors the herbs that Carolyn had been taking to help with PMT and stress. They seemed interested, but unconcerned about natural herbs having any effect on her heart, although I did get the impression that alternative medications were not their preference.

❧

Monday morning brought me a new challenge. Dave and CJ were leaving. They had responsibilities back home, and Carolyn seemed out of immediate danger. So they bid farewell and took the hotel shuttle to the airport. Just before he hopped on board the bus, Dave handed me the rental car keys.

"Do you remember how to get to the hospital?" he asked with a wicked grin.

I was alone again in a foreign city, within an even more foreign country, driving a strange car on strange roads, trying to get a grip on the frightening event that had brought me there. With my heart racing as I retraced the relatively simple route from hotel to hospital, I felt like a candidate for cardiac failure. At least I was headed to the right place!

I had not noticed before that the hospital was located next to highway 114. It was weird that this gave me some comfort. There is a route 114 that leads right into the street we lived on in Salem, Massachusetts. I was acutely aware of this because I had only just begun driving around on my own with confidence. After all, every time I took the wheel, my instincts told me I was driving on the "wrong side" of the road and sitting in the passenger seat!

Navigating the roads in Massachusetts is a test of one's mental faculties, and perseverance is required if you want to get to your destination. It seems that each city or town wants to keep you within their boundaries, and so they have avoided signposting important intersections and junctions, to prevent you from leaving the town—lest you forget how to get back! New England is such an old part of the country, that these roads could have been walking tracks and leaving town was rare, even if it was only a few miles. But surely, now, they could put up a few signposts, and choose better roads to have as main arteries!

Having safely negotiated the broad and well signposted Texan roads, I parked the rental car in the enormous parking lot, and made my way down the now familiar corridors, noticing for the first time there were new spectators to the endless drama in the emergency ward. It was a little sobering to realize that there could be more patients in critical condition when I entered the ICU. Passing by the waiting room I saw some familiar faces and said hello. One lady asked me how my wife was doing and I replied that she was now awake—good news is always well received.

Whoever said they don't like Mondays? When I asked the ICU nurse on duty how Carolyn was that morning I was stunned by her answer. Carolyn had improved so much that there was talk of her leaving ICU that afternoon! The other nurses were as amazed as I was; this was virtually unheard of. Usually the only patients to leave ICU within a few days are deceased!

Chapter 5

PLUMBING FOR ANSWERS

*The art of medicine consists in amusing the patient
while nature cures the disease.*

—Voltaire

No longer sick enough to warrant the close supervision of an ICU ward, Carolyn was still in need of hospitalization. Her heart had stopped functioning a few days earlier, and her lungs had been given the equivalent of a severe beating, so she desperately needed to rest. She had been transferred to the cardiac recovery ward and was now sleeping peacefully in a room with a view. The room was enormous, with a sofa under the window that suspiciously looked like it could fold out as a bed. Sure enough, I checked with the nursing staff and found that we had been given a room for two! They told me the ICU nurses had specifically requested I be able to stay with Carolyn due to my positive effect on her vital signs.

Carolyn was still only sleeping fitfully, and when she awoke, I shared with her the news of my new accommodation. She bounced up and down on the bed with glee, but then clutched her chest in agony. The sudden movement had pulled on the cardiac monitor leads and patches stuck all over her ribs, which were extremely sore. It was nice to see a return of the happy little girl I knew, even if it was only fleeting. She lay back and smiled at me, such a warm and welcoming sight in such an austere place.

I decided to check out of the hotel, and brought all our clothes to the hospital room, so I wouldn't have to leave her alone anymore. It also meant I didn't have to drive back and forth the five or so miles everyday, and could spend all the time with my gorgeous wife.

In the process, I took the opportunity to get some creature comforts from the shopping mall down the road. My hurried selection of clothes from home suited Boston weather better than the Texan fall, and I needed some lighter, cooler apparel. I also wanted to get something to brighten the room, now that Carolyn was conscious and able to appreciate it.

We still didn't know how long we would be there. The weekend had passed without further advice on her affliction. We did know that there were more tests required, but little in the way of detail. I got the distinct impression that we could be there the whole week before an answer would be forthcoming.

Carolyn had had calla lilies in her bridal bouquet and wandering around the huge warehouse of a store I found the perfect arrangement. It was so well made it looked real, even down to the faux water in the bottom of the vase! I knew she would be pleased to have a vase of white lilies as a reminder of our wedding the month before. The lilies had made such a statement of beauty and grace, and I could picture her sitting up in the morning and, seeing the sunlight fall on the lilies, be able to escape the harsh reality of where she was and why. I could certainly have used a distraction as well.

I had not realized that Carolyn was gaining enough strength to start causing havoc with the hospital protocols. Returning from my shopping expedition, I entered the nursing station and sensed some tension—a foreboding in the air. Previously, when I walked in there would be smiles and hellos tossed about. This time, however, no one looked my way, and Carolyn's assigned nurse did not make eye contact with me—he almost ignored my arrival. I had felt quite comfortable leaving Carolyn with that kind and caring male nurse, so what could be wrong? As soon as I entered her room I could see that there was indeed a problem. Carolyn was fuming and ready to bite anyone that came near her.

"What's going on?" I asked, not seeing anything wrong with her physically. In fact she looked almost normal to me, so there was obviously no medical issue. One part of me liked what I saw—maybe she was "all better now" and her collapse was just a false alarm. Reality contradicted this dream. Only a few days ago, she had been clinically dead, her pupils had been "fixed and dilated" which implied that the brain stem was cutoff, and *that* could not be ignored.

"I won't have these unnecessary procedures. These American doctors are always over servicing their patients; that's what's wrong with the health care in this country!" she said, her jaw set and her eyes dark and grey, instead of their normal hazel color.

The nurse had unwittingly provoked that fire and tempest I knew so well. We may have only recently married, but I had known this wonderful girl for several years, during which she had shown her passionate side more than a few times!

I held back my initial reaction to the outburst, and attempted to "seek first to understand"—the 5th principle of Stephen Covey's *Seven Habits of Highly Effective People*. This performance improvement program has techniques that apply to nearly every misunderstanding or conflict. We had learned to use the principles at home even more effectively than at work, and I was now hoping to use them to avoid any more stress for Carolyn. And the rest of us.

So what was the problem? What could that diligent, competent male nurse have done that sparked this distress? He had only asked Carolyn to sign a consent form for the angiogram procedure scheduled for the following day.

"I had a complete check up by the cardiologist in Australia last year, and there was nothing wrong with me. They do not need to do an angiogram," she stated.

I calmly waited for her to continue. There was more to this than meets the ear, I sensed.

"Do you know that they are very dangerous? I used to work in a radiology lab, and there were always problems with angiograms!" she explained. She then bit her bottom lip, and looked at me a little sheepishly. But her eyes looked wary, ready to flare again.

I was glad I had restrained myself. An irrational fear had jumped up and bit us—that would teach me to leave the room. "Yes, darling, it *is* a dangerous procedure. They will put a catheter into the femoral artery in your leg, and thread it all the way up into your heart. But it is very common now, and they need to see what is wrong with the arteries feeding your heart," I replied gently but firmly, and being careful not to sound patronizing. I was hoping to diffuse the situation so we could stay on the surgical schedule, since not checking the condition of her arteries was unlikely to be useful in determining the problem with her heart.

Before long, Dr. Preston, the resident responsible for Carolyn in the cardiac recovery ward, strode in to talk to us about the "heart-cath" procedure. He tried to make Carolyn calm down and understand the importance. It took him well over thirty minutes to convince her that despite the previous tests in Australia showing no heart damage, it did not explain why she went into V-fib a few days earlier.

In other words, whatever the condition of her heart a year ago, it was different now!

Carolyn could not win the argument, and I suspect she knew it, but she wanted to have her opinion heard. I was definitely supportive of the doctor's intention to continue with the procedure the following morning. We had to find the cause; she couldn't possibly leave the hospital otherwise.

Carolyn accepted this reasoning, but not without the last word. "I want you to tell them to talk to my doctor in Australia. He can tell them that there is nothing wrong with my heart!" She looked ready to leap out of bed and do it herself.

I agreed that it was a reasonable request, having her past history could be helpful, especially her cardiac records. So, close to midnight in Dallas, I found myself sitting at the doctors' station (it was just a bench with a few PCs and lots of medical texts strewn about) searching the World Wide Web for a specific cardiologist in Melbourne,

Australia. I had to find a phone number, or better yet an email address, so that Dr. Preston could discuss the patient records from last year with Carolyn's cardiologist in Australia. Amazingly this was all possible with the Internet, and within an hour I had the required details. Dr. Preston contacted the Australians and by mid-morning he had received the information he deemed relevant.

The Australian cardiologist had dismissed Carolyn's original complaint as a benign cardiac arrhythmia, after they had done a chest x-ray, echocardiogram and had made her wear a Houlter monitor for twenty-four hours. None of those results helped Dr. Preston, and I think he had suspected as much the previous evening. The reports did not explain why Carolyn had suffered a cardiac arrest, nor did they indicate that she was susceptible to an arrest. It provided him no new information at all. The angiogram scheduled for the next day was the only definitive test, and it could identify the cause.

ᦞ

An angiogram is an examination of the blood vessels using x-rays. It is an invasive procedure that can determine if there are significant coronary artery blockages, and allows planning of angioplasty or bypass surgery. It would be performed by inserting a catheter, a long plastic tube about as thick as a strand of spaghetti, into Carolyn's femoral artery in the groin and guided through the arterial system into her heart. The iodine contrast agent, a substance that x-rays cannot pass through, would then be injected into the blood vessel so that images could be taken of her coronary arteries. Carolyn was right about the risks, but serious complications or death occur less than one in a thousand procedures. The catheter could damage an artery or loosen a piece of plaque lining the artery wall, and this loose piece of plaque could travel up the artery to her brain and block the blood flow, causing a stroke.

The procedure was to be performed in a cool and sterile catheterization laboratory that resembled an operating room with monitoring devices, video display equipment and x-ray cameras. The camera is called a fluoroscope, or C-arm; a large arc shaped piece of

109

equipment that generates x-rays from one arm above the bed and photographs them underneath, displaying the results on a CRT monitor in real-time.

I was told it would take a few hours, and was introduced to a volunteer who could guide me through the whole nerve wracking exercise. The friendly, elderly chap explained that he had had an angiogram prior to his bypass surgery. I'm not sure which of us was more surprised that there was such an age difference between us, but I was impressed with how slim and fit he was. It was my first experience of the apprehension and hope associated with a loved one undergoing a serious operation, and I appreciated his kind words of advice.

ℬ

Carolyn had only just recovered from the sedation when they wheeled her back into our room. I felt sorry for her. She had been doused with drugs again, and those terrible tubes and wires had returned. When would these invasions of her body stop?

Since her femoral artery had been pierced during the procedure, a special collagen plug (called a VasoSeal) was inserted into the hole to speed the body's natural clotting process. The plug was covered in clear plastic wrap that stuck to her skin, preventing any stretching that that could cause the wound to leak. In addition, Carolyn had to lie quietly in bed with her leg held straight for six hours, to make certain the plug sealed properly. Otherwise, she might bleed to death!

ℬ

Dr. Hecht looked at me with a slight tilt to his head and said, "I now understand how she survived ten minutes of CPR. Her arteries are in perfect condition, and she has excellent blood flow." He handed me a glossy printout of her heart, showing two views of the blood vessels feeding her ventricles. The arteries were picked out by the dye, and looked like the fine roots you see when transplanting seedlings into pots.

I nodded, and looked down at the photo of Carolyn's heart. Okay, so now you don't think she has had a heart attack? Furthermore, she has nice clean pipes, and there will be no need for the medical equivalent of "Draino".

"So what does that mean then?" I asked. Instead of being relieved or grateful, I wanted to know where that left us. In the back of my mind I was aware that I was behaving in an "I told you so" manner—a bad habit of mine. And none of us had listened to Carolyn. She had been right all along, there was nothing wrong with her coronary arteries!

"It must be the electrical system," he said. "We need to have her undergo an EP study. That's an electrophysiology test, which can check the electrical pathways in her heart muscle, and show us where the problem lies."

"I see. And then?" I asked, wondering if we were getting any more certain of what was wrong or still searching for possibilities. Ruling out the plumbing was a good result; no need to open up her chest and fiddle about with her heart. I had read about stents and angioplasty, where clogged blood vessels are propped open with a fine mesh tube inserted into the artery, a procedure that is similar to the test she had just undergone, but that had never been mentioned as a probable cure. It seemed we didn't need to consider that solution. I was now being led towards the unknown again, and the hope that an EP study would uncover the problem with Carolyn's heartbeat.

"She will probably need an implanted device." Dr. Hecht sensed my bewilderment, and backed up a little. "I can't say for sure, but I have a colleague who is very experienced in this field, and I'm arranging for Carolyn to be transferred. He will decide what needs to be done."

"An implant?" I could not believe he was serious. What sort of implant I wondered. Surely Carolyn doesn't need a pacemaker!

"Yes, the chances of her surviving when this happens again are very slim. You should not consider leaving here without a safeguard. She probably needs an Implantable Cardioverter Defibrillator to stop the deadly ventricular fibrillation."

It was my turn to look at him piercingly, "This will happen again?"

"Statistics show a likelihood of one in three that she will have another episode in the next two years, and the survival rate is less than five percent." His tone indicated there was no negotiation. No choice. No alternative scenarios. An EP study followed by a device to protect her from a deadly repeat episode.

These Texan doctors were certainly giving it to me straight. First, they told me she was in critical condition, next that she had had a heart attack, and then I was told that whatever it was, it was highly likely to happen again!

～

That evening Carolyn and I discussed the passage of another day without a clear prognosis, and wondered when we could be sure of her future. She was nonplussed by the results of the angiogram; after all she had vehemently tried to tell us that there was nothing wrong with her arteries. But the specter of an electrical problem did scare us. Wasn't that called an arrhythmia? Had the benign become malignant? I'd heard the term benign used in relation to tumors, meaning it was "safe", not progressive, or not dangerous to health. But, it didn't sound right using the same term for a heart problem.

Dinnertime interrupted these thoughts, and there was little point in deliberating on them anyway. We were not the experts and had little or no say in the matter. Carolyn's appetite did not stretch to the bland and texture-less meatloaf and vegetables presented on a sturdy plastic dish that had seen so much use that it was battered and scuffed all over. A nasty side effect of the oxygen she was required to breathe through a tube under her nostrils, was that everything smelt like a gas leak and tasted metallic. She was interested in the salad and of course the applesauce pudding. So I ate the protein and starch while she had the carbohydrates and sugars!

A tall thin man, dressed in slacks and dark shirt that was open at the neck, sauntered into the room and stood at the end of the bed. He said hello to no one in particular and peered at the clipboard in his hand. He looked up at Carolyn in expectation. I knew that he was Dr.

Solomon, the neurologist, and felt critical of his manner. He was so abrupt and almost dismissive. He could have been friendlier, or at least polite. I watched very much as a spectator while he put Carolyn under deliberate emotional stress. I couldn't help thinking that he must be lied to often, since his demeanor was just like a policeman's—distrusting, until you prove yourself.

"Do you know who I am?" This first question was fired at Carolyn in a very aggressive way.

I was little alarmed that he appeared to be checking to see if she remembered him at all. Was there going to be bad news following this examination? Did he suspect something I had not seen or noticed?

I could see Carolyn bristle at his arrogance, but she answered calmly, "You're the guy who tells me if I have brain damage." What a comeback! I was so proud of her frankness, it reminded me of that evening in Sydney when I was first smitten. She could be so forthright and direct that I had been totally disarmed—she captured me so.

He continued on, wanting to know where she was. "In Dallas, on a conference," was the pert reply.

"What happened to you?" he probed.

"I had a cardiac arrest." This time she faltered and the tears welled up in her eyes.

He did not pause. The questions came barreling out. What day is it? Where do you live? Where were you staying? When did you get here? How did you get here? Do you know the name of the hospital? On and on he went. I could see that soon he would hit that defiant streak in Carolyn. I suspect she inherited it from her mother, Helen. When those eyes harden and glint, you want to watch out. I had learned early on in our relationship not to try pushing Carolyn on an issue, stopping before she got that "Don't tell me what to do" look. At times, I would tease her by asking how old she was, and what it was that she really wanted, because her defiance was almost comical in the way that it emulated a four year old. I could almost picture her as a little girl, stamping her feet, saying, "No, I won't." My teasing often drew this out, and was a reasonably successful technique to defuse the situation, but not always advisable!

I was intrigued to see how this professional "brain doctor" would handle the impending outburst.

"Why are you asking me all these stupid questions?" she demanded with a tilt to her head and a hardening of her lips.

I wanted to step in and rescue the situation. I could see by the look on the neurologist's face that he did not know her well enough, and was ultimately just trying to determine her mental faculties. But I kept quiet and, sitting on the chair beside the bed, leant forward to look carefully at Carolyn's face. I knew he was going to hit her limit soon, and felt compelled to stop him. I began to nervously shift in my seat.

Dr. Solomon pushed on regardless, increasing the stress level by firing back his reply, "Because I need to determine your neurological status. I cannot sign your release until I have diagnosed you."

My compulsion to act was too slow, and I watched as Carolyn struck back with a masterful retort to the interrogation. "Well I happen to know that humans only use around three percent of their brain capacity, so if I have lost some memories or functions I'll just have to learn them over again! I don't think you need to treat me this way!"

Unperturbed, but with a trace of a smile at the corner of his mouth, Dr. Solomon explained that he needed to check her ability to recall long-term memories and whether she could build, store and retain short-term memories. Brain damage can often be identified if there is a hesitation or confusion about memories, especially short term ones.

Now, Carolyn was worried—I could see it in her eyes. She *did* have memory problems. She couldn't remember what happened—how she got to Dallas, or even the tube that had been in her throat. She knew there had been a tube because her throat was so sore, and she could hardly talk above a whisper (and now had a wonderfully sexy, husky voice). She was still angry with him, but her professional instincts had kicked in. She didn't think he had been handling the consultation at all well, and wanted to tell him so.

Despite Carolyn having more to say, she couldn't sustain any more talking, so she wrote her questions out on my notepad. *"How long does this take? I think you should let people know what to expect because it is traumatic."* She turned the pad around so that Dr. Solomon could read the words, but she didn't receive much in the way of acknowledgement.

"I am a teacher. I always seek feedback for improvement. You don't have to agree," she continued with an emphatic punctuation mark, the pen nearly penetrating the paper.

He did not seem affected in any way, and told us both that there would be one more consultation the following day. He also said that Carolyn seemed to be recovering well, and then he turned around and left the room. Just like that, the examination was complete.

I was nearly overwhelmed by this development. Despite the odd manner, it seemed that he was going to clear her of any neurologic problems. Carolyn did not seem to appreciate this. Understandably she was still annoyed, and more than a little confused with the abruptness of his departure, so I explained what I had just witnessed. After a few minutes, she conceded that it may indeed have been a test, and that she had passed with flying colors. After all, she had retrieved a long-term memory about the capacity of our brains, and her short-term recollections were accurate, although understandably not complete. And we hadn't even told him that she'd also been able to remember the name of her Australian cardiologist!

But she wasn't really convinced. In reality she was confused and frightened about her arrest, for which we still had no explanation.

"I don't remember the tube! Memory loss!" she scrawled, followed by a renewed bout of crying. Her eyes were wide open and her mouth contorted, the tears rolled out as soon as they were formed, and she looked around the room as if searching for something. I had seen this look of frustration before, and it was often followed by desperate anger, so often the reaction a powerful person has when they cannot control

their environment. Had I spoken too soon? Was there really no brain damage? How could we be sure? Only time would tell, and I did not mind waiting this time. I really didn't want to know at all, as she seemed so normal now.

I held Carolyn tightly and gently rocked her back and forth, agreeing with her that the situation could be better. She was slowly accepting that a very serious thing had happened to her, that she had been heavily sedated for several days and still had the after affects of drugs and hypoxia. I wanted her to let the perfectionism slide, and just go with the flow for a while. She relaxed in my arms and went to sleep. The effort of talking just those few minutes had drained her.

While I felt that Carolyn's condition was improving, I knew she had not yet recovered from the horrid effects of the cardiac arrest. Still under constant supervision, she was alive, but for how long? Would she arrest again? Could the wonders of modern medicine really unravel the problem, or would this be just another one of those "interesting cases" where the patient unfortunately couldn't be saved.

Was I being impatient, or even unrealistic in my optimism? When would the doctors find out what was wrong? I was becoming frustrated, and yet I just had to wait to express my feelings some other time. Right then, I had an important job to do, and that was to ensure my gorgeous girl was looked after, and was as comfortable as possible.

Chapter 6

THE ELECTRICIANS

Doctors are men who prescribe medicines
of which they know little,
to cure diseases of which they know less,
in human beings of whom they know nothing.

—Voltaire

The hospital phone beside the bed rang, startling us. Who knew the number? We certainly didn't and hadn't given it any thought, with cell phones being almost the exclusive technology now. We were lying together on the narrow hospital bed. Carolyn had finished her uninspiring evening meal, and we were talking quietly about what little we knew of her collapse and its cause. This was a common subject, and Carolyn raised it at least once an hour, if not more often, depending on how long she slept. If she had a long sleep the question would come up fairly soon after waking, but with some of the shorter naps she was able to remember the earlier conversation. She could never remember enough to carry on where we had left off, so we covered the same ground over and over again. The ring had emanated from a phone attached to the bed head. I fumbled with the curly cord, catching the handset before it fell to the floor, and answered hesitantly, tilting the earpiece so Carolyn could hear as well.

"Hi, this is Dr. Wells. I am an electrophysiologist at Baylor Hamilton. Dr. Hecht has referred me, and I want to talk to you and Carolyn about the EP study." It took me a few seconds to realize that "EP" stood for electrophysiology.

"Yes, Dr. Wells. We have been told that another test is necessary, and that it will help detect the electrical disturbances in her heart. But we've not been told much else," I replied. Carolyn still had a weak, hoarse voice, and wasn't ready to engage with yet another doctor.

The call started to sound faint and scratchy, and he stopped his car to continue. He explained some of the technical aspects of Carolyn's case and seemed confident that he would be able to determine the cause of her cardiac arrest. Then his voice changed, and we heard the frustration push past his calm professionalism.

"There is a problem with your insurance company. Apparently they will not authorize the procedure. I am furious that our hospital administration could not sort all this it out earlier. Do you know anything about this?"

"No, but I have been learning about HMOs and their rules. Is there something I need to do? I thought that this was automatically covered as an emergency," I replied, with a sense of foreboding. I sensed that arranging the PCP selection with the HMO several days earlier had been a very good idea after all.

"Well it is, but technically the transfer to another hospital closes that claim, and the EP study and subsequent implant could be classed as elective."

"Do we have to change hospitals? Couldn't we stay here?" I asked, thinking that this was a little too obvious a solution.

"Maybe I should explain," he replied, and continued on for several minutes, outlining the special laboratory required, and the complex procedure to measure the heart's electrical pathways. While Baylor Grapevine did have sophisticated cardiac surgery capabilities it did not have an electrophysiology catheterization lab, and thus, Carolyn would need to be moved to the new Baylor Jack and Jane Hamilton Heart and Vascular Hospital, downtown. He reiterated the danger of not having a device implanted, and that the electrophysiology test was necessary to determine which device would be best and how it should be programmed. This was delivered in that same non-negotiable manner I had heard in Dr. Hecht's voice. Were cardiologists continually dealing with clients who don't want their services? Or, like the neurologists, are they just suspicious of a patient's motives? I suspect that denial is a common factor for all their patients, and has to be dealt with swiftly and early in the conversation.

"I have Carolyn scheduled for the test on Thursday morning, but we need to have her admitted tomorrow." He paused. "Don't worry about the insurance issue, I will personally ensure it is resolved." Another pause. "But, I do need you to guarantee the charges in order to get you into the schedule." The calm professionalism had returned, and my salesman's instinct was alerted. He had overcome the first barrier—we did have medical insurance—and he was now swiftly moving us to the "close".

I hesitated for a moment, and asked, "How much are we talking about?" The discussion had moved a little faster than my limited experience with hospital charges allowed.

"Well, probably around fifty thousand dollars. But I'm sure you will not be required to pay. I understand your wife works for IBM and I'm certain they will be able to help you straighten this out. I want to have her admitted tomorrow, and the personal guarantee is a formality our administration insists upon, I'm sorry."

Carolyn and I looked at each other as he finished. I could see she did not want to deal with this decision, but I was loath to commit to such a large amount without her understanding. We had transferred sufficient funds from Australia to get established in our new country, but not for surprise medical expenses. I had heard horror tales of U.S. medical costs wiping out a lifetime of savings, and those stories now had a hard reality to them. Surely, this was just a bureaucratic wrangle. We had medical insurance and she was on the job when her cardiac arrest occurred, so there should be little likelihood of our actually having to pay.

Carolyn looked away in disgust that a patient would have to consider such a circumstance, having spent two decades in a country that considers health care an essential service, funded by the taxpayer.

I put my hand over the telephone microphone and said to her, "You have excellent medical insurance, and Jim will help if it comes to a fight. We don't want anymore delays, do we?"

She accepted my reasoning that it was a calculated risk, and nodded to the phone in my hand.

"We can guarantee that amount so that she can be admitted, but I am not agreeing to the procedure at this point, okay?" I said to Dr. Wells.

"I understand, Mr. Whitehead. I expect it will be resolved, and you shouldn't have to pay. I'm sorry for asking. I am furious with our administrator, it should never have come to this." He paused but I said nothing, and so he continued, "I'll make the arrangements right now to transfer her tomorrow."

And with that simple statement, we began the next step in our education of the miracles of the human heart. We knew that Carolyn's plumbing was not the problem. Now, we were to face the shocking world of electrophysiology. Would that be the end of it? And what ending would it be?

૭

After several more complex phone calls the next morning, the insurance issue was settled, and it was time for Carolyn to see a little of the Dallas metropolis. She was to be taken by ambulance, as in fact, she was not being discharged, only "transferred" to another ward, albeit nearly twenty miles away!

The preparations for moving a cardiac patient appeared to be almost the same as for handling an emergency. Carolyn had to wear an oxygen mask, and a portable ECG monitor was attached to the patches still stuck to her chest. In addition, the defibrillator was charged and ready to go. The ambulance men were actually EMS technicians, and equipped to deal with an arrest if it should occur in transit. Carolyn slid over onto the ambulance gurney and they lowered her down to knee level, but they did tilt the back up so she could see were they were going. I gave her a kiss goodbye, and said I'd follow in the rental car.

"Will they turn the lights and siren on?" Carolyn asked me, since she had missed it the first time. She was so cute in the manner of a little girl asking for a treat, reminding me of one childhood Christmas when my cousins had asked my uncle if they could go for a ride in his police car, "with the lights and siren on?"

As we walked down the corridor to the elevator, I asked them where we were going, and explained that I was not familiar with the roads. The EMS guys said I could follow them so I wouldn't get lost, and to meet them out front.

I walked over to the ambulance to check that they knew which car I was driving. The driver smiled at me and said, "I'll try to stay under eighty, but ya'll can't follow if we has the lights on!"

He did stay under 80mph, but only just! It was unlikely I would lose them—that big red, blue and white truck speeding down the multi-lane highway, with a silhouette of Carolyn in the back, sitting up and taking in the view through the tinted rear window.

When we arrived at Baylor Hamilton in downtown Dallas, I was tempted to follow the ambulance all the way into the emergency ward loading-bay. Instead, I parked in the street and hurried over in time to catch them before they were swallowed up in the bowels of the huge University Medical Centre.

Just as I arrived at the rear of the van, the driver caught my eye and said, "Yo wouldn't believe how many people follow us right in here. Yo lucky yo di'n't." His grin was wide enough to show the quality of his dental insurance.

They already had Carolyn out, and had extended the wheels on the gurney, ready to wheel her away. Not sure what to do, I followed the ambulance men through the emergency ward, down a corridor and into an elevator. They had instructions on where to take Carolyn, but the wing had only just been completed, and no one knew exactly where we had to go. Eventually we were led to a catheterization lab, and I followed the gurney through the swinging doors into a prep-room. Everyone in the room was wearing surgical gowns and caps, and they turned to look at us. Carolyn, sitting up on the gurney at chest height, had a commanding view. The look of horror on her face must have surprised the technicians more than her unexpected arrival. They soon recovered and continued with their activities, but not a word of complaint was heard.

In a plain matter-of-fact way, the EMTs were told that Carolyn was not on their schedule, and that we must be in the wrong section. Once they sorted it out, we were given some complicated directions to get to the correct ward.

And what a ward it was. Wood paneled walls, plush carpet and Dell flat screen PCs were on every desk. It looked more like a business office than a medical institution. A swarm of nurses in royal blue jumpsuits took over, and Carolyn looked like the queen bee as they deftly settled her into our suite. And I mean a suite! There was a sofa bed for guests, an en-suite with shower, toilet and vanity, plus a double wardrobe, bookshelves and a stunning view of the Dallas city skyline. Was this the real reason the insurance company had balked at covering the EP study?

❧

Mark had arranged yet another hotel room for me, in the same complex, but on the other side of the hospital gardens, a few hundred yards away. That meant I got a little exercise, walking between the hotel and Carolyn's room twice a day.

While I had willingly given up the previous hotel room, I was now suffering from sleep deprivation. I had made a tactical error in deciding to move into Carolyn's hospital room. Every couple of hours the night-shift nurses had waltzed in, turned on all the fluorescent lights, noisily checked her pulse and blood pressure, taken a blood sample, or given her some medications, as per the orders on the chart. I, of course, was abruptly made aware of all this activity, and tried in vain to blot it out with blankets piled over my head.

While I gladly accepted the break from living in a hospital ward, there was an additional benefit; Carolyn showed such excitement each morning when I came over, it was like the first time, again and again.

I had been grateful to have the rental car during the first week, but now that we were downtown I wasn't planning on going anywhere and it seemed a waste to leave it at the hotel unused. So once Carolyn was settled in, I invited Mark to visit and that evening we had a little adventure in the Dallas city streets to return the car to Hertz. Mark and I had a chance to talk as normal people, and it was a nice escape for me to hear about his family and all the dramas and excitement of living with small children. I was sure he would have preferred to be with them, instead of escorting a hospital ward zombie who still had no answer to Carolyn's collapse.

જ

One of the first health professionals we met in this new hospital was Tracy, the Respiratory Care Practitioner. I joked that he was a Sammy Davis Jr. look-alike, but one of his major assets was an uncanny ability to find the veins in Carolyn's arm. Whereas nearly everyone else had a devil of a time and ended up sticking her multiple times, causing unnecessary pain and concern for Carolyn, Tracy had the touch, and was done before she noticed he had even begun.

"She has a central line, why don't you use that?" I asked Tracy, concerned about Carolyn's arms again, since they had just started returning to a normal color and texture.

"We have a policy not to use IVs that we haven't inserted," Tracy answered. "But this triple lumen catheter is in good condition. They must have flushed it regularly. I can use it for the blood draw," he continued almost apologetically.

"She had it put in at Baylor Grapevine, you know." I felt like arguing, but I could see there was no point; I had no power or control in these minor medical matters. His need to put a new IV into Carolyn's arm was probably the least of our worries.

"She is not likely to need any drips here, and we only put the IV in as a precaution," he smiled, a genuine smile that disarmed me immediately. "We have to take that central venous catheter out anyway, if she is going to have an implant, you know."

"Fair enough. How come you can get it in first time every time, no pain, no fuss?" I asked, pointing to the new IV line in Carolyn's arm and hoping my previous irritation didn't show.

"Yeah, I'm known around here as the best IV man, with good fingers," he replied, surprisingly happy about the reputation and wiggling his wondrous digits in the air. "There's nothing wrong with her. Even though you can't see them, she has perfect veins; they're just below the surface. You simply have to feel for them!"

He then showed me how to gently touch the top of Carolyn's forearm, and close my eyes to help me feel the vein, like a soft tube or drinking straw just under the skin. He told me that even though you cannot see the blue vein, you just have to trust your fingertips and insert the needle in exactly that spot—apparently it works every time. Not that I would know, I've never done one!

Tracy was not there to insert IVs. His job was to evaluate a complication with Carolyn's lungs. She had an infection, probably caused by aspiration during the CPR, and they wanted to clear it up fast. He immediately requested a portable, upright chest x-ray, to diagnose her "productive cough", as they feared she might develop pneumonia. This was to become a regular morning event, but we didn't know that at the time.

&

Having only just become familiar with the layout and services available at Grapevine, I was now thrust into a new environment. The path from Carolyn's ward to the hotel bedroom was as confusing and tortuous as below decks in a battleship or cruise liner. I had to navigate subterranean tunnels, identically colored corridors and sub-floor elevators. I'm sure I never took the same route twice, and had wished I could have taken the stairs instead.

In order to retain some form of control I quickly established a routine. After waking and showering I would spend half an hour or so eating a delicious BLT sandwich and a coffee in a café downstairs. I relished watching the rest of the world go by before having to face the confinement of the ward. Despite the plush décor, it was a hospital room and Carolyn was being attended to just like in the ICU. No peace and quiet, no privacy, and little to do but talk and worry.

Time moved so slowly in that sumptuous suite. Like waiting for the train home at the end of a workday, each minute seemed like six hundred seconds, not sixty. I had lost connection with the days of the week, and resolving hours in the afternoons was nearly impossible, for that was the quietest time in the ward. It reminded me of siesta time in Italy, when nearly all the stores in the village shut up shop and the piazza becomes deserted. In the hospital, there was a solid block of three maybe four hours with no interruptions or activity until the evening mealtime, after which there was the doctor's rounds and meds to be administered.

❧

Baylor Hamilton Heart and Vascular hospital is integrated into the University Medical Center and features nine interventional catheter-ization and electrophysiology labs, with some of the most advanced digital imaging technology. That was why we were there—to find out what was wrong with Carolyn's cardiac conduction pathways. She needed an EP study. They would be mapping the electrical system that caused her heart to beat, but from inside her heart! This involved inserting another catheter, into a vein this time, to stimulate another cardiac arrest and measure her heart's electrical impulses on a computer screen. The analysis of those electrical signals, and the tests for abnormal rhythms would then provide the data for programming the device that Dr. Hecht had suggested would be necessary.

I found it chilling that this controlled death was to be performed around ten o'clock that Thursday morning. It was exactly one week earlier, almost to the hour, that Carolyn had suffered a cardiac arrest, and they had unwittingly chosen the "anniversary" to make it happen again!

What was most frightening was that her precious heart had to be stilled as part of the test. I hardly felt prepared for the responsibility of consent, or the dread of its ramifications. Dr. Wells was as insistent as Dr. Hecht had been, and their reasoning was unequivocal. It was vitally important—her life depended on it!

Carolyn was wheeled away to the electrophysiology lab, where she was to have yet another bout of sedation. If Dr. Wells could recreate the precise electrical stimulus that had caused the arrest, she would need to be defibrillated again. I found it hard to accept that he was going to try to kill Carolyn, stopping her heart with a small shock, delivered at just the right time and in exactly the right place. For those dozen or so seconds she would be dead; there would be no pulse, and no life giving oxygen for her brain and organs. To ensure he had achieved precisely the right conditions, her blood pressure and heart rhythm would be monitored. We were assured Carolyn was not going to feel any pain, or suffer in any way.

But we *had* been asked to provide an advance directive, just in case anything should go awry.

Anxious to know what Dr. Wells would find, I was also scared about what might go wrong. I had no option but to wait in our suite for Carolyn's return. Unlike the angiogram there was no volunteer to help me through this procedure, and it was lonely waiting for her to come back. I hadn't experienced the vacuum of her absence since she had left home for Dallas a week earlier, and I empathized with how she must have felt when I went back to my hotel room each evening. I started to feel depressed.

I needed something to do. I noticed the phone socket on the wall and wondered if I could use Carolyn's laptop to get onto the Internet. Maybe I was just suffering web withdrawal; it had been over a week without getting online. Until that moment I had treated her company ThinkPad as an extra piece of luggage, albeit an important and valuable one. But once online, I was amazed to find more answers to my worries and anxiety than from the live experts in the hospital.

After that first foray on my own I got into the habit of dialing up every time Carolyn slept, to check out the medical sites. I learned how to communicate more effectively with her surgeons, accumulating their terminology and becoming familiar with their technology. I can honestly say that without the Internet, I would have been totally lost. It reinforced the power of the web as an essential learning tool. I was also able to read my email and realized that I had not cancelled all those appointments I'd made with potential employers. I had no idea when we could return to Boston, or whether I would be able to continue my job hunting.

It seemed that every time I found a respite from the isolation and uncertainty I faced, the realization of the severity of our position crashed through. I felt my sphere of influence close in again. My focus narrowed to just Carolyn and her wellbeing—nothing else seemed relevant. I had one task, that original task, to take her home. To recuperate. Then I would be able to think about the future.

⤳

Dr. Wells is a medical professional, with clean, quick motions. His small, dark athletic build exudes an aura of speed, and his manner is focused and functional. So when he walked into the room still dressed in green Operating Room garb, facemask dangling with beads of sweat still on his brow, I sensed he was not pleased. He had difficulty maintaining his Mr. Fixit, can-do approach.

"We tried everything, but I had to give up." He looked at me from under his brow and shook his head. "We could spend hours testing and still not find the ectopic foci that caused the arrhythmia. Oh sure we could induce the fibrillation, but that's all." Again he gave me that look. "There was no point putting her under any more stress. I tried everything, atrial and ventricular overdrive, ventricular extrastimuli...." He paused to see if I was following the technical mumbo jumbo. "We did get a few beats of AV Node Reentry Tachycardia, but nothing sustained."

I did not sense that Carolyn was in any danger; rather, he was annoyed that he was unable to find problem with her heart.

"And that's not good?" I asked, even though I had followed most of what he had just explained, a result of my investigations on the web and reading the HeartWise patient education pamphlets he had given us the previous day.

"Well no, I wouldn't say that. It's just I hate not finding anything to point to the cause of her arrest. Carolyn still needs to be protected, the results of this test don't rule that out." He shook his head in irritation again and said, "She has an idiopathic deadly arrhythmia." He looked me in the eye. "Which means we can't determine the cause."

After furiously writing on the chart, he continued, "Carolyn should be back in here shortly, she is still recovering from the anesthesia. We'll proceed with the ICD implant on Friday." Finishing with a sharp stab of his pen on the chart, he looked up and seeing the panic on my face said, "I'll come by later to introduce you both to my colleague Dr. Wheelan, who will assist in the operation. We shall talk about the operation in detail so you will know what to expect."

I cannot say that we were expecting anything in particular, other than an explanation of why Carolyn had suffered a sudden cardiac arrest a week earlier. Dr. Hecht had been incorrect in his presumption that Carolyn had blockages, and now Dr. Wells could find no definitive proof of her "faulty electricals". But along the way, we had somehow accepted that a device would be the final solution.

By this time I had read enough to know about the danger and effects of ventricular fibrillation, but what about the cause? Would it really happen again? How could they be so sure, if he couldn't find the specific cause? I felt trapped in a non-negotiable position.

It was too dangerous to risk another episode without protection. A prophylactic measure was Dr. Hecht's term. But why should it occur again if there was no fault to be found in her heart?

Hadn't Carolyn's reluctance prior to the angiogram been verified? Was this another example of the "unnecessary medical procedures" she had objected to? She had been correct in saying there was nothing wrong with her heart, at least on the plumbing side. And now, it seemed there was nothing tangibly wrong with her electrical system.

∾

Dr. Wheelan was tall and charming, with a calm and quiet nature. He seemed concerned, and despite his almost formal and reserved manner, he was genuinely interested in helping Carolyn deal with the apprehension of undergoing an implant procedure and its repercussions. He explained what an ICD was, paying particular attention to how the technology had advanced from the large, bulky, short-lived devices that required extensive surgery with multiple incisions, to the high performance, small and long-lasting units now available, that can be programmed to respond to specific arrhythmias.

We were sitting together on the edge of the bed, listening to Dr. Wheelan finish his pitch on the virtues of modern medical technology, when Dr. Wells turned the discussion toward the best placement of the device. We had read the brochures, with their graphic depiction of the device placed in the chest, under the collarbone, so we knew the basics. He began by explaining that they would not place it under the pectoral muscle as the trauma would take longer to heal and the titanium case could rub against Carolyn's ribs. Then, Dr. Wheelan outlined how the electrode lead would be inserted into Carolyn's subclavian vein, just near her left armpit, and fed into her right ventricle. The lead is screwed into the heart muscle to ensure a good electrical contact, and to hold it in the right place. The other end of the lead, where it exited the vein, would be permanently sewn into place. But the device would sit in a pocket cut into her flesh, because it would need to be replaced when the battery ran out. In the process of these revelations both doctors touched the respective parts of Carolyn's body, as though she were a dressmaker's mannequin.

"I think we can hide the scar under your bra strap, and you should not see much of a bump," Dr. Wheelan said to Carolyn. "Just here I think, don't you Dr. Wells?" Dr. Wheelan had his index finger hovering over the slight depression under Carolyn's clavicle, just above her left breast.

"Yes, she is quite delicate, but I think you're right," Dr. Wells replied. "It should not show, especially once the capsular tissue binds to the implant. We can make the stitches narrow, and the scar nearly vertical so it will not be visible in anything other than a bikini."

The dialogue would not have been out of place at a bespoke tailor; put a seam here, let it out a bit there. Carolyn and I looked at each other and wondered about a shocking little computer implanted in her chest; ready to go off at any instant. I knew the surgical corrective action for faulty plumbing could be frightening, but the outcome these two medical electricians portrayed was plain scary!

॰

The wound in Carolyn's chest from her central line was healing slowly. Unfortunately, it was in the same place as the pouch they needed to create for her implant. In addition, she still had a bad cough, and the infection in her lungs was deemed serious enough to delay the operation. Dr. Wells didn't want Carolyn coughing during surgery, and there was little consensus about the hazy x-ray images taken each morning. Was there solidification into a firm dense mass or not? He recommended postponing the operation to Monday or Tuesday so that the infection could be cured and to give the wound more time to heal. Dr. Wheelan concurred.

We would just have to wait. Again.

In the meantime, Tracy had a special therapy to help clear Carolyn's lungs—what I called her peace pipe. This was a corrugated plastic tube with a mouthpiece at one end, and a bottle below, containing a liquid that turned into a wispy vapor as she sucked in the air. She had to take big breaths to get the medicine deep into her lungs, but this was very painful. The nurses had explained that it was to be expected; the CPR would have stretched the cartilage in Carolyn's sternum, and possibly bruised her ribs. But the vapor would make her breathing easier, if only she would suck it all the way in!

Anticipating that the end to this nightmare was nigh, I decided to checkout of the hotel. I wanted to spend all my time with Carolyn, and could use the sofa bed under the window in that sumptuous suite. I did not think there would be the same degree of interruptions in the middle of the night as we had in the ICU and cardiac recovery ward at Grapevine. At least, I hoped not.

Besides, now that Carolyn was able to communicate and hold a normal conversation, we could start to plan our return to Boston. I was eager to get out of Texas and take my poor sick girl home. The end was now in sight and she looked alive and well, compared to that disastrous sight in ICU when I had first arrived in Dallas.

On each morning of the previous three days, we had received a special delivery of lush plants and flowers sent by Carolyn's colleagues and relatives. The vases and baskets filled all the bookshelves and overflowed onto the windowsill. All those beautiful blooms and get-well cards made the suite so bright and cheery that it was hard to imagine that ten days earlier Carolyn had been near death in the sterile and harsh environment of an ICU. Carolyn was touched that even colleagues she had not properly met at the conference had sent their best wishes. It was another demonstration of the IBM family sentiment we had never noticed before.

ଈ

I could tell that Carolyn's cognitive functions were improving when she began to get annoyed with the late-shift nurses. There was a fold-out whiteboard on the wall at the end of her bed, and every evening these night owls would bustle in, rub out my three standard answers to Carolyn's perennial questions—what, when and where—and write, in large letters, their name and the cut off time for dinner orders. Carolyn glared at them and yet said nothing to stop this aggravating behavior. I sensed that she resented them taking over and changing her world but she lacked the energy to complain, and since we never saw the same night nurse twice, she would have had to repeat the complaint every evening! It was a small sign that she was concerned about controlling her domain, but I felt that it was an important indicator of her mental health. At no time prior to this had she been concerned about her surroundings, or the nurse's activities. Unless it had something to do with her bodily fluids of course!

Carolyn had the occasional legitimate complaint in the first hospital, and while not easily communicated, they were usually easy to solve, predominately relating to her physical discomfort. Now, we were facing situations where her will was greater than her ability, and the frustration was clearly evident. At times, I found it difficult to tolerate her demands, and should probably have expected some friction arising from such a strong willed person. While I was perplexed by the tension, I was also thankful that she was a fighter. She may not have recovered from the arrest without that determination.

Before long, these frequent instances of annoyance, bordering on anger, and often towards me, led me to wonder if Carolyn had begun the process of grieving. She had every right to; she was now brutally aware of the fragility of life. She had died, but it must not have been her time, so she was destined to linger with the living, shocked and unsure of her future.

Whether Carolyn was going through the stages of grief or not, I was sure she was suffering the loss of her purity and innocence in heart problems. If she had thought she was not afflicted like so many of her family, she could no longer make that claim.

The time had come for us to discuss the ramifications, and what changes the implant was going to have on our lives. Carolyn was scared and very unsure of the future. She was even more frightened that she was now "damaged goods", and that I might think less of her. She was also anxious about being unable to continue her work. I think we both subconsciously leapt over the possibility that she could still be in danger. Not because of our trust in the device or the doctors, but because admitting the threat was to accept that we no longer had complete control of our lives. I was not ready for that conversation. Perhaps I was the one stuck at that first stage of grief: denial.

Whenever these thoughts and fears threatened to upset me, I reminded myself that there was a valuable service I *was* able to perform. Carolyn did not have to face this nightmare alone. I was right beside her to help, as decision maker and interpreter, and she relied on my cognition, as hers was still impaired. Some decisions were simple and enjoyable, like helping choose her meals each day from the menu, or reminding her which tablets were which and what they were for. Carolyn also wanted me to recount the details of her collapse. She wanted to be able to remember what had occurred, and hoped that hearing me describe the actions and reactions of Tom, Randy, Jim and her managers would trigger her memory. She also needed help in accepting the need for an implanted device. I am not sure I was the best person for the job, but I tried my best to interpret the technical aspects, and patiently listened to her emotional outpourings. Actually, I was having trouble with my own disquiet about the device, so listening to her voice those fears was beneficial.

Carolyn had actively listened to the doctors, but I could tell she had not fully appreciated what they were saying. At times, she had looked into the distance and I could see her mind switching off in self-protection. She was not ready to face the fact that her heart had failed, and that she needed a "gizmo" inside her to stay alive. I could hardly believe it myself, and yet we were forced to brutally face this major life-altering decision.

"What did he say I have?" Carolyn asked when she noticed I had packed up the laptop for the day. She was sitting upright in her bed, and had been woken a few minutes earlier when that evening's night owl burst into the room to do her thing on the whiteboard and check the blood pressure and pulse. We had already phoned in the dinner selection, and Carolyn had a full pitcher of water on her side table, so there was nothing more for the night nurse to attend to and she left us alone.

"Idiopathic. But that just means they don't know!" I replied. I had been eagerly searching for a reference on the web, since I couldn't accept that all those tests and procedures had resulted in the statement "…we can't determine the cause." According to one site I found, approximately five percent of sudden cardiac deaths have no demonstrable cardiac or non-cardiac causes to account for the episode, and are thus classified as idiopathic ventricular fibrillation.

When I first heard the word used, I had considered idiopathic an idiotic diagnosis, but then I thought the term might not be so bad after all, and could be used to our advantage. I decided to share the thought. "Darling, maybe 'idiopathic' is good—not knowing means that it is possible we can beat it. Whereas knowing the cause might mean it is unavoidable and something is definitely broken or faulty."

The logic may not have been sound, but it seemed to offer hope. Carolyn just looked at me in silence, and then looked away. I don't think she saw anything promising in the diagnosis, nor the solution. I did not share the fact that while looking up that obscure word I had found another more confounding term—iatrogenic, which is doctor-speak for "it's our fault". More accurately, iatrogenic means induced inadvertently by medical treatment. I decided that word did not need to be a part of our vocabulary.

We were facing that terrible choice misfortune presents: do you hope some new information may come along that indicates things are not so bad, (that a miracle might even occur), or do you believe that all the options have been identified and the outcome is final? We had all weekend to consider the question, and come Monday we would just have to be ready.

Meanwhile, the rest of the world continued to struggle forward, to which Carolyn was oblivious. A creature of habit, I usually listen to the news every morning on the radio, read a good newspaper once a week and watch the TV news every evening. But for over a week I had no interest in world events, nor the local issues and scandals. I didn't even know what the weather forecast was, so consuming was my melancholy. Consequently, we did not know that the Senate Debate on Iraqi WMD, which resulted in Congressional authorization for the "use of force against Iraq", had occurred while Carolyn was unconscious. And the terror bombing in Bali on October 12, 2002 also went unnoticed, despite the ghastly deaths of seventy-eight of my countrymen, with over two hundred poor souls dying in that massacre.

We had our own private war to worry about, conquering the deadly arrhythmia and banishing it from our lives. We could not have it threatening our freedom, fearing it may strike at any moment—that unannounced and hasty serial killer.

Chapter 7

A SHOCKING DEVICE

*Medicine, the only profession that labors incessantly
to destroy the reason for its own existence.*

—James Bryce

The comment kept drumming in my head like a mantra. "It would be the best thing to do, as a prophylactic measure, you understand?" Dr. Hecht had said a week earlier. What could he have been talking about? We had no need for prophylactics; we'd been practicing safe sex, and each had had only one partner for several years aforetime. But he wasn't concerned about our sex life.

He had been leading me to the realization that Carolyn needed an Implantable Cardioverter Defibrillator, an ICD. It would be like having a paramedic with her at all times, constantly monitoring her heart rhythm and ready to correct any abnormality within seconds. She needed that prophylactic protection—insurance against the devastation another collapse would bring.

Maybe I should have one too? I could be at risk of a sudden cardiac arrest, although the statistics didn't support the concept. If I did suffer an "episode", I would most probably die, yet another inconceivable death. A terrible loss to the community, unavoidable and such a shame, "He just dropped dead; a perfectly healthy, fit, young man," they would say. I would not be alone. There were the celebrated sports stars like Reggie Lewis, a 28-year-old Boston Celtics basketball star, who died in 1993 shooting baskets; or Darryl Kile, the 33-year-old St. Louis Cardinal's baseball pitcher who collapsed and died in his Chicago hotel room in 2002. I'm no longer a teenager but they, too, are vulnerable; Adam Lemel was 17 years old when he died during a school basketball game in Milwaukee, Wisconsin. Project ADAM (Automatic Defibrillators in Adam's Memory) was created in his name to provide automatic external defibrillators (AED) in public places, particularly in schools. And even Vice President Dick Cheney could have joined this ignominious list of preventable dead—because his cardiologists determined him to be at high risk of sudden cardiac death after surviving his fourth heart attack. He now lives with a state-of-the-art ICD in his chest.

Unfortunately an ICD is not a cure, it is purely a protective device, and the only guaranteed protection available all day, all night wherever you may be. There was never any discussion of carrying an AED about with her everywhere, hoping that a Good Samaritan would be willing and able to operate the device if Carolyn arrested in public. In the early 1980s, I once worked with a fellow who had a deadly asthma condition. He carried a suitcase containing an oxygen bottle and syringes with powerful drugs, in case he had an attack. We were expected to follow the clear and precise instructions on the suitcase lid—otherwise he would die. Luckily he never collapsed at work, although his wife had had to use the dreaded suitcase several times at home. Maybe Carolyn is more fortunate than him, in that her solution—an ICD—can be implanted, and she doesn't have to expect strangers to use an AED if she collapses.

Dangerous heart rhythms like ventricular fibrillation are usually irreversible, and can only be halted by a high-energy electrical shock. Drug therapy alone is unable to rectify this abnormal rhythm and, for the foreseeable future, pharmaceuticals are regarded as inferior for the treatment of sustained arrhythmia events. That is not to say that drugs are of no use, it is just that they cannot stop the chaotic rhythm once it starts. They can reduce its likelihood, and are very useful in assisting the recovery process.

Carolyn will always be at risk of the deadly arrhythmia. Since there is no known cure, and drugs cannot terminate the deviant electrical impulses, we had to accept the shocking solution. It will be implanted "forever", this tiny digital computer with on-board memory and precise programming. The microprocessor and battery are contained in a smooth, shiny titanium shell that is not much bigger than a stopwatch, and ought to be unobtrusive under the skin below her collarbone. It would be connected to the muscle inside her heart via a special insulated and flexible electrode, called a lead, which permits both monitoring of the heartbeats and delivery of the electrical energy to restore a regular rhythm. Since medical technology is developing rapidly and the battery has a finite life, the device will need to be replaced every decade or so. So, "forever" really means forever having an operation to reinstall a new unit!

When the heart starts to quiver instead of contract, a tremble replacing that strong and regular beat, it is useless for the purpose of circulating blood. With ventricular fibrillation, there is an electrical signal of sorts, but it is chaotic and faint. The individual ventricular muscle cells contract in spasms, not in unison like a well-practiced orchestra. Anarchy rules, and the ventricles hardly squeeze at all. The sinus node, that natural pacemaker of the heart, fires and the atria contract, attempting to push blood into the already full ventricles. The electrical signal is supposed to then be delayed a fraction of a second by the AV node which will trigger the ventricles to contract powerfully, expelling the blood into the aorta and the pulmonary arteries. During V-fib, however, the ventricles do not respond. An external electrical signal is required to repolarize the cells. The body uses only a few joules of energy to maintain a normal sinus rhythm. An external defibrillator typically can deliver over three hundred joules, since the paddles are placed on the outside and have to overcome the resistance of the skin and bone of the chest wall to reach the heart muscle. Despite having a direct path to the heart muscle, an ICD may be programmed to deliver over thirty times the power naturally consumed by the heart. That is substantially less than an AED, but it is still a powerful shock, and more than enough to restart the heart; but not so much that it will cause the body to jump, like an AED can.

"Will it hurt?" was the first question Carolyn had for Dr. Wheelan when he stopped by on Saturday morning to check there were no "developments". I recalled popping into the office on weekends myself, just to tidy up those few loose ends left over from the workweek, but I hadn't considered that for a doctor that would mean visiting a patient.

"Well you will certainly know it has gone off!" he replied. The attempted humor did not provoke a response from Carolyn. "Sorry, no, I shouldn't think so, you would most likely be unconscious. And there wouldn't be any of the soreness you feel now from the CPR, nor would there be the burn marks you have from the paddles." These words did register, and Carolyn visibly relaxed. So pain will not be a factor in the "therapy" she may or may not receive from the device. Unfortunately, I could not help Carolyn adjust to this horrible reality, other than being by her side, holding her and listening. I understood the technology and some of the medical aspects, but I could not fathom the fears and worries of actually having a thing inside my body that was designed to zap me without warning.

Dr. Wheelan continued in a more formal manner, probably sensitive to Carolyn's unease, but also eager to reassure us both. "You will be scrubbed down and have an antiseptic wash applied early on Monday morning. I have ordered some Valium to help you with the anxiety; it should also take the edge off the pain in your sternum." I was surprised he remembered, as Carolyn had not complained to him directly about the sharp stab in the chest she received every time she coughed. But then, that cough had delayed the operation so he was definitely aware of it.

Carolyn was not talkative, and I felt the time was not right for me to ask the hundreds of questions I had. Was it the engineer in me seeking a way to assimilate the news? If I had all the specifications, the physical dimensions, and understood the programming parameters, could I give her the support she needed? Should we not have all the facts? How could I accept the inadequacy of my knowledge and experience in this momentous decision? Did I have any right or authority to intervene?

I decided to follow Dr. Wheelan out into the corridor before asking him which manufacturer and what device they had selected. At least with that information I might be able to quell my own reservations; to investigate online and glean all the technical details I sought. Unlikely as it seemed, I had already found online discussions of ICD "owners" regarding the various shapes and sizes of the three major manufacturers products. There were also ominous descriptions of devices going off repeatedly. And yet, all these strangers' comments ended with gratitude toward the device, as without one they could be dead!

Until that point, I had not felt that I was able to contribute very much to our discussions on implants and the "shock therapy". But using the research talents I had developed as an IT marketing executive, I soon became absorbed in uncovering a wealth of information on the subject.

I was surprised to find that electrophysiology is the fastest growing field in cardiology, and that it is a fairly recent discipline. Technology has done much to advance the field, but it is no wonder the Food and Drug Administration did not approve ICDs until 1985, five years after the first human implant. That first generation device was only able to terminate arrhythmias that exceeded a given rate by delivering fixed high-energy shocks, and it required open-chest surgery to attach the electrodes. Second-generation devices gained programmable output and backup anti-bradycardia pacing. The third generation ICDs introduced the internal lead technology and enhanced programmable features. Fourth generation devices are smaller, and combine dual-chambered pacing, defibrillation, and leads with expanded sensing capabilities. Eventually, ICDs will provide combined monitoring, recording, and treatment of any type of rhythm disturbance, and other cardiac complications such as acute myocardial ischemia.

I learned that Medtronic, the manufacturer of the device Carolyn was to receive, has nearly twice the market share of the other two device manufacturers, St Jude and Guidant (now owned by Boston Scientific). All three produce other medical devices but the ICD market alone is a multi-billion dollar industry. Medtronic is the largest of the three and was founded by Earl Bakken in 1949. I was intrigued by the similarities between the worlds of Information Technology and medical devices. Reminiscent of Hewlett Packard, Bakken started Medtronic in a garage, with his brother-in-law, as a hospital equipment repair company. By 1960, they were producing pacemakers and were fortunate to be pioneers of Minnesota's innovative medical device industry, sometimes known as "Medical Alley." That was more than two decades before we all learned about the infamous "Silicon Valley" on the west coast. The company is now proud to state that every six seconds, somewhere in the world, a person's life is saved or improved by a Medtronic product or therapy.

Guidant Corporation pioneered ICD therapy by developing the first implantable defibrillator in 1985 and call their units AICDs which stands for Automatic Internal Cardiac Defibrillator. They also claimed to have the world's smallest, thinnest dual-chamber ICD— that senses both the right atrium and right ventricle to detect a wider range of abnormal rhythms. (Unfortunately the Indiana based company had a technical problem with their PRIZM device in 2005, and soon after they merged with Boston Scientific.)

St. Jude Medical started making mechanical heart valves in 1976, but twenty years later acquired Ventritex, Inc., a California based ICD manufacturer. Their claim to fame was the Atlas+ HF ICD, apparently the most powerful ICD offering cardiac resynchronization therapy— using small shocks to re-coordinate the action of the right and left ventricles.

I found peace and comfort in learning about the device Carolyn was to receive, and gained insight into how it would be connected to her heart, and why. We had been frightened that the reason for her collapse was unclear, and that it could happen again. But my rudimentary education, courtesy of the abundance of medical information on the web, helped me gain understanding and comprehension of the science involved, the mechanical designs and solutions, and the certainty that knowledge brings—the confidence that Carolyn would be all right after all. It reminded me of the 1970s TV show *Six Million Dollar Man*—"we have the technology, we can rebuild him". Except there was no rebuilding required, just a small addition; an enhancement; a private cardiac rescue robot.

Carolyn had appreciated my technical prowess in the past and I expected she would be interested in my findings. She knew my habits, but I was surprised that just knowing I was doing the research emboldened her. She didn't want the details, only my verification that having the implant was a sensible thing to do. She relied on me to sort out the complex terminology and unravel the mysteries of cause and remedy. I felt useful and worthwhile, not just a spectator. I finally had something to contribute.

And yet, what we found most valuable were the personal stories and discussions about experiencing the life-saving shock from an ICD. Somehow reading about other people, who had similar issues, and how they faced them, helped us accept the inevitable. Carolyn would be joining this group of lucky and permanently altered survivors. And we were learning to be thankful that she would always be protected against the deadly arrhythmia that had threatened our wonderful new life.

೨

At last, we were coming to the end of our nightmare in Dallas—at least the physical side of it. Carolyn had survived *three* cardiac arrests, two of which had been deliberate and controlled. Finally, she was protected against any future episodes. Three arrests in two weeks had given her body such a beating, and yet most of the abuse was in the form of a medical cure.

On a Thursday morning in October, Carolyn's heart had spontaneously contracted ventricular fibrillation. She was remarkably lucky to have willing and able bystanders keep her alive until the EMTs could revive her. It was many hours before she stabilized that first time. And then a week later, almost to the hour, she had to die a second time. The only difference being, this time she had been *scheduled* for the repeat episode. An electric shock stopped her heart, not an errant beat. Only a small shock, but it was delivered at just the right time and in exactly the right place. She was dead; there was no pulse, and no life giving oxygen for her brain and organs. Her blood pressure and heart rhythm monitors showed the precise conditions had been achieved. She was sedated, so she did not feel any pain.

Three days after that, Carolyn had her third arrest. This time the device was in place and ready for its "maiden voyage". It fired its first jolt of electricity directly into her heart muscle, just as it was designed to. Connected to the electrodes only a few minutes earlier, it was programmed with specific parameters unique to Carolyn. Again, a short, sharp shock was used to make her heart begin the deathly twitching. Within seconds, her newly implanted computer detected the abnormal rhythm and waited until the capacitor was fully charged. A few more seconds passed as it checked the rhythm again, and without further delay it delivered the restorative thunderbolt. That first discharge used up about two weeks of the battery's life.

I did not get to see it, and neither did Carolyn. I know the place where "it" is, that foreign metal object that pokes into her ribs when she crosses her arms, or rolls over in bed. But I was not permitted to touch the lump, or allow my eyes to linger too long on the scar. *It* is hidden inside her, constantly monitoring, waiting for the chance to run its program, prepared to charge up and then deliver the climatic discharge, only to start waiting again. Just like *The Terminator* it is a machine—and as Kyle Reese, the character from that Schwarzenegger movie, warns, "it absolutely will not stop."

❧

Carolyn now has to accept the fear of "*it* going off", not just the surprise kick in her chest, but more from the realization that if the device were not there, watching and waiting patiently, she would most likely be dead. Carolyn would probably not be aware of this "therapy" since the ineffective pumping of her heart would cause abrupt unconsciousness, if only for the few seconds it takes for the shock treatment to be delivered. She could be driving and crash the car, or walking on the street and fall down, or maybe she would be sitting down and just slide off her chair like that first time. She may even be asleep and be woken by the sudden thump. It is unlikely that I would notice, even lying in bed beside her.

Carolyn doesn't like pain, and prefers to avoid it at all costs. She was neither prepared for, nor able to escape the pain and restricted arm movement that came with this implant. It had immobilized her. Like a winged bird, only half her body was functioning properly, and she wasn't able to perform simple basic chores. She couldn't lift her arm above her shoulder and so washing her hair, getting dressed or even tying her shoelaces were impossible tasks. She was now forced into behaving like a child, but through disability, not personality.

Nevertheless, I reveled in her dependence upon me. I had not had that obligation to another person before, and I relished the opportunity to care and provide for her. I was enjoying the responsibilities of being a husband.

I did, however, feel ill-equipped to confront what we both feared most. Neither of us was able to address the overriding question. How would this bump under her skin affect our lives?

One particular comment from one of the many websites I visited on those long afternoons, struck a chord with us; "Inevitably, ICD patients have to confront significant lifestyle restrictions, or possibly contend with psychological problems."

Yes, we *would* have to confront changes and deal with the emotional scars, as well as the bright red blemish of the fresh wound under her collarbone. The stitches were neat, and designed to fall out when the skin had healed, so there was no need for a follow up visit.

We were free to go!

Weeks of waiting and now, just like that, Carolyn was "fixed", and was discharged the next morning.

Chapter 8

LEAVING DALLAS

Do the hard jobs first.
The easy jobs will take care of themselves.

—Dale Carnegie

We had finally arrived at the task I had originally prepared for in Boston. I was bringing Carolyn home. Could it have been only two weeks earlier that I had left Salem? It seemed to have taken much longer than that to find the remedy for her surprise medical emergency. But then, almost without warning, we were facing the prospect of leaving Dallas. After so many days of uncertainty and indeterminate testing, the countermeasure was installed on Monday morning and we were to be gone the next day!

Carolyn's final journey from the suite at Baylor Hamilton was not the first foray on her feet, vertically aligned and under her own power. We had taken two tours of the ward over the weekend; with Carolyn gripping the IV stand on wheels like a drowning swimmer clinging to a lifesaver. She had been trembling, whether from feeble muscles or a feeble mind I couldn't say. I showed her the kitchen where I had made my morning coffees and the refrigerator with the little boxes of cranberry juice she had so often requested. We passed an examination room with its special table and cabinets full of utensils and dressings. Then we came to another suite that was not as big as ours, but was otherwise the same. A frail old lady lay on the bed, and she had several visitors who had a petrified, frozen look on their faces. I wondered if I, too, had had that appearance?

The first walk left Carolyn bushed after traveling only fifty yards, and she needed to lie down to regain her strength. The second time she made it all the way around the ward and felt masterful enough to get a drink from the kitchen by herself. The freedom and feeling of self-sufficiency did wonders for her outlook. My wife had begun to emerge from her ordeal as healthy and normal person again, if only she could get out of that hospital gown!

Going home, however, was suddenly threatening to be a stressful event, not the happy occasion I had anticipated. Carolyn was as weak as a kitten, and just as loveable. She could hardly walk a lap of the ward without requiring a sleep afterwards, and her left arm was now in a sling. She was glad to be rid of the hospital gowns and had begun to feel like a real person again. Despite wearing the comfy clothes I had brought from home, Carolyn was not feeling comfortable at all. Her shoulder was throbbing and her ribs were still extremely sore from the CPR. The skin on her chest and neck was tainted yellow from the antiseptic scrub, and the fresh wound had large bruises forming, probably caused by the pocket cut into her chest for the device.

We had been warned that the device could set-off metal detectors and I recommended that we not endure the rigmarole of airport security, especially considering the post 9/11 paranoia. Air travel was becoming intolerable for healthy non-metallic people, with all the bag inspections and clothing removal.

How could Carolyn possibly cope with those demands? She was supposed to be recuperating.

My first class ticket had an open return date, and Jean, Carolyn's assistant in Boston, offered to investigate alternative travel arrangements. Carolyn and I had discussed taking the train, reasoning that a leisurely overnight train-ride was preferable to the hustle and bustle of airport concourses, especially with the drama of finding a wheelchair and passing through security with an implant.

"How long will the train take?" I asked Jean, remembering that Carolyn and I had traveled to Providence on a very fast train, called the Acela Express, during our first trip to America in 2001.

"Well, Amtrak doesn't go directly from Dallas to Boston. So there are actually two trains you would have to take."

Jean eventually explained to me that our options were limited. We really only had two choices: a six-hour flight, if you include the interminable airport delays and time zone change, or three days by train.

Three days! This was obviously not the Acela Express.

We decided to take the train. A bed, three square meals a day, and the chance to cuddle; versus being strapped into an airplane seat, struggling with a fold out tray and turbulence? The choice was easy, and I suggested we treat it like a holiday. I'd not seen much of the country and the Amtrak route would take us straight through the heartland of this abundant country to Chicago, the windy city. We would then head East past the Catskill Mountains through the middle of the Empire State. The Berkshire Hills were next, and finally we'd be back home in Boston. If we were lucky we might catch a few "trees on fire", although the best of fall had been and gone while we were enjoying the enforced southern hospitality.

౭

Despite the practice laps around the corridors, Carolyn was not allowed to walk out of the hospital when discharged. The nurses insisted on bringing her down to the car in a wheel chair, and they were nonplussed that we weren't expected to use it after that! It was just another education in the side benefits of American liability insurance. Was she only permitted to fall down outside the hospital, not inside? Luckily the platforms at Dallas Union Station were relatively easy to access, unlike Penn Station in Manhattan, but not as straightforward as those at Boston South Station. A short walk down, and then a ride up in the elevator put Carolyn almost exactly at the carriage door. We had a sleeper car, and the conductor was kind enough to give us a cabin on the same level as the dining room so Carolyn wouldn't have to negotiate the stairs on a moving train.

There were more surprises in store for us. Similar to the luxurious hospital suite, the sleeper car had its own shortcomings. It was situated at the front of the train, and little did we know that the train was required to signal its advance at each and every railway crossing. Regardless of the time, whether it was three in the morning or three in the afternoon, the engine driver blasted the countryside with a long and piercing wail from the horn, to frighten any and all road traffic from entering the intersection. He was highly successful; we didn't hit anything, and most of us were awake to verify the fact!

Luckily, we had been conditioned to sleep deprivation by the regular and insistent nursing routines over the previous weeks. At least being woken by the horn was less intrusive than having the fluorescent lights turned on for Carolyn's blood pressure and temperature checks. I wouldn't say we missed the attention and dedication of those night owls, but I did sense that something was missing. Carolyn's reaction to leaving the hospital came as a surprise to me. She told me she didn't feel safe outside the ward, without the heart monitors and medical personnel just a few seconds away. Not fully confident that her heart was going to keep up its strong and regular pumping, she was anxious that she might not be so lucky a second time. I reminded Carolyn that she had her own private EMT crew with her at all times, literally on her shoulder watching her every minute of the day. I told her that she was perfectly safe, and that the ICD could do a quicker and better job at restoring her heart to a normal rhythm than any external force. My words were received cognitively, but emotionally they were ineffectual. It had not happened to me, so I could not appreciate the terror of feeling perfectly healthy one minute, and waking up in intensive care the next.

The residual effects of Carolyn's cardiac arrest were going to take some time to dissipate.

We just had to wait. Again.

৵

Our cabin was comfortable and cozy, not as salubrious as the hospital suite, but at least there weren't any nurses to barge in on us. It was inevitable that Carolyn would need to raise the up-to-now avoided subject of what had happened to her. She also needed to rationalize her new bionic addition.

"You can't live without a heart, and yet mine is faulty," she said to me abruptly, as though I had been reading her mind.

"And darling, you have an ICD now, so you aren't in any danger," I replied without missing a beat. Voicing her fears was excellent therapy and I wanted her to continue. She looked down at the floor and bit her lip. She seemed unconvinced that *it* would make a difference.

"I trust the device, but what about my heart?" She finally replied. "It's not normal, and they haven't been able to find out what is wrong with me!"

It was clear to me that Carolyn wanted to be reassured. I didn't think she was "damaged goods", but I had to help her come to the same conclusion. We spent many hours discussing her crook heart and the conversations always included the bump above her left breast. Occasionally, she would pull back the collar of her shirt to inspect the damage. A scab was forming over the stitches already, but her skin was badly bruised again. The dirty yellow stain of antiseptic scrub was giving way to the yellow tinge of fresh bruising. Soon it would start to turn a hideous mottled blue-green, and then vivid purple, as Technicolored as her arms had been. Her left pectoral muscle was very tender and sore, and she could not lift her arm at all, which made dressing quite difficult and washing her hair impossible. I, however, was eager to assist.

There had been little opportunity for us to be intimate in the hospital. Cuddles had not been physically possible, and Carolyn hadn't seemed able to be affectionate in any case. Inside the train cabin, with the door locked, we were finally alone; no interruptions, no monitoring, and Carolyn was free to move about. After two weeks held captive in bed, and constantly having fluids removed—sometimes voluntarily, and at other times rudely awoken at the appointed hour—Carolyn was distinctly pleased to have finally regained control over her physical life.

I was also pleased that we had the privacy; there was something we had talked about several times but not yet had the opportunity to pursue. Carolyn had had little inclination to consider anything more than the lowest levels of Maslow's hierarchy of needs: the physiological and safety needs. Was Carolyn now ready to explore the higher levels: love and esteem?

Carolyn was obviously feeling very fragile, but also needing the physical comfort only a partner can provide. We had escaped that harsh clinical environment where bodies are abused with drugs and procedures, and now wanted to explore the pleasures of the flesh, not the pain. I felt like a virgin again, awkward and fumbling like the first time, unsure where to touch and what to do. It was an exquisite feeling, and almost worth the anguish of those past few weeks.

Carolyn's skin was soft and warm, her senses heightened by the lack of touching, and she shuddered as I kissed her gently on the neck, just between her jaw and right ear. I, too, shuddered, but I could feel us melting into one another, my shoulder sliding into the gap between her bicep and ribcage, my arm curling around her waist, my legs entwined in hers, and my eyes greedily scanning the curve of her cleavage. Her breathing became shallow and quick, and I was still holding mine; we both felt the anticipation, but also the fear. She was not ready; she was still adjusting to that foreign body under her skin. The combination of sweet and sour heightened our senses. Mixing a little tension with desire had created a powerful aphrodisiac. I deliberately slowed the pace—thinking, "let her drive the agenda here buddy, just stay 'north' a while," as Dr. John Grey advocates in his relationship books. She kissed me more passionately, more insistently, as we squeezed each other tighter, wanting there to be no barrier between our bodies. I looked into her eyes, and saw her desire. She saw my restraint and relaxed. I desperately wanted her to let my caresses be more intimate. She surrendered to my passion and I unclasped her brassiere, sliding the strap off her good shoulder. Neither of us looked at the other shoulder, we just left it hidden and forgotten.

I tasted her smooth luscious skin, glowing in the moonlight cast through the trees, flickering as the train sped through the night. Her eyes pleaded: hold me, take me, and be gentle. I felt her soften with the waves of pleasure. We were quickly intoxicated. Lying together in the moonlight we both realized that Carolyn was the exactly the same person I had married less than two months earlier. We were feeling the love, not the scar tissue, and coming through this calamity in more ways than one!

A tear escaped and rolled down her cheek. It tasted salty and I was reminded of our first time in Australia when Carolyn had asked me a very leading question. "Is this love?"

With typical male chauvinism, I had attempted to avoid the topic and replied, "I think it's ecstasy!"

We still talk of that moment and relish my instinctive words. Both of us do. For ecstasy was exactly what we had achieved in our relationship, and the little scare Carolyn had given us in Dallas made it all that sweeter.

It would always be ecstasy for me.

Chapter 9

MIRACLES

Something was dead in each of us,
and what was dead was Hope.

—Oscar Wilde

Centuries ago, bringing back the dead required divine intervention. It was a miracle no mere mortal could perform. Notwithstanding his studies on the "furnace of life" and the vital spirits, the ancient Greek physician Galen concluded that there was no possibility of rekindling the innate heat provided by the heart. Throughout the Middle Ages it was widely believed that death could not be reversed; the furnace of the heart was lit at birth and extinguished at death. And yet, despite the advances in medicine, and more importantly emergency care, the odds of surviving a sudden cardiac arrest in the twenty-first century are less than one in ten. Where you live, where you work, and how you travel to and from work all impact the likelihood of survival.

There are two fundamental survival tools required. The most important one is free, and is nearly universally recognized—it is called CPR. When you are on the brink of moving from the quick to the dead, mouth-to-mouth resuscitation and chest compressions can stop the clock. If, however, your heart crosses that fine line between vibrant and dormant, and you approach the edge of darkness, a defibrillator will be the only solution. Every hospital has one, and you're probably already aware of their "crash carts". Hardly any of the medical dramas on television fail to have those ubiquitous paddles in use. And yet defibrillators are relatively rare pieces of safety equipment, much as fire extinguishers once were. Often the first responders are not equipped with one, and not all public buildings have them either, although there have been hundreds of thousands of units manufactured in the US alone. How many more need to die before these revival devices become ubiquitous? Do you know where to find one right now? How soon would the EMTs arrive with one if you had a cardiac emergency at this moment?

Today, we recognize that divine intervention is not necessary, but a miracle is still required to save someone from sudden cardiac death. And yet the miracles do happen. Carolyn was in the right place at the right time. Was it because the angels were watching over her? Who can say? She certainly has a recollection of angels, but that was probably after the miracle, once she was in the safety of a hospital intensive care unit.

It was a miracle that there were bystanders willing and able to sustain her life force, right at the time she collapsed. The cities in America with the best bystander CPR rate can only achieve a one in two chance of the victim undergoing CPR by the time the rescue crews arrive. Dallas wasn't one of those cities. Was it a miracle that both Tom and Randy were CPR trained and experienced, and right there in the room? Perhaps the American Heart Association, Red Cross, Atlanta police force and the US Army should be acknowledged as contributors? The AHA and Red Cross are attributed with the successful education and promotion of CPR. Carolyn certainly benefited from Randy's police training and experience, as well as Tom's military service. Without performing CPR within a minute or two of her collapse, the chances of brain damage would have been great, and the progression to permanent death might have begun. Her survival was really only possible because the EMTs carried a defibrillator as part of their equipment. Would Carolyn have survived if a different class of ambulance had been dispatched? Not all emergency services have defibrillators, and even if they do, not all the vehicles are equipped.

Perhaps it was a miracle that a nurse, Kathy Williams, heard the commotion and went to help, assisting in the CPR and encouraging Tom and Randy to continue when they may have stopped.

It was certainly a miracle that Carolyn's arrest occurred when there were people nearby—not when she was in the shower, walking down an empty corridor, or sitting in the back of a taxi coming from the airport. (She was probably safer in an airplane because the FAA ruled that they be equipped with AEDs since the turn of this century). Carolyn could have been just another statistic in the fight against sudden and unexpected death. After all, only one in twenty victims are saved. Who were those unfortunate nineteen that did not survive? Why is it that Carolyn was not one of them? What possible reason could there be for my beautiful bride to have beaten those horrific odds?

It was a miracle that a top ranking hospital was located just five minutes away. The EMTs were skilled in resuscitation, but they were not equipped to prevent abnormal heart rhythms, and could only provide a temporary solution. An AED can restore a normal rhythm, but it cannot protect against another episode. Carolyn did relapse into cardiac arrest—after the EMTs had resuscitated her—in the emergency ward. Intensive care was required, and the time in between was critical to her long-term survival.

It truly is a miracle that Carolyn suffered no brain damage after enduring more than ten minutes without normal blood flow. The statistics mandate that only two or three percent of victims will survive that long without oxygen and a pulse. What made Carolyn so special that she could beat those odds as well? The angiogram showed remarkably clear arteries, so there was little or no restriction to the blood flow for her brain, heart and lungs. But CPR is not nearly as effective in providing circulation to the body as a properly beating heart, and is unlikely to sustain a reliable blood pressure. As Kathy Williams said after I had called to say Carolyn was home and safe, "Well she beat all the rules and statistics—it is miraculous."

Divine intervention may not be required to resuscitate a victim, but seeking solace through prayer has been constant and widespread throughout history. Prayer seems to be a natural and instinctive urge—to communicate with the Almighty and "ask for assistance"—yet it is not accepted as a certain remedy. Perhaps God decides the fate of a victim, and prayers can only help guide that decision.

Had a higher power decided that Carolyn has more to do? Was her purpose in life not yet complete? Could it have been the prayers? There were nearly a dozen different groups of people in four different states all praying for Carolyn's health and safety. Some could be heard in the ICU, others were just a few miles down the road at the Hotel, but the majority of these wonderful people were thousands of miles away. From Atlanta to Boston and Rhode Island, they participated in a multi-denominational intercession.

Prayer offers so much to so many people and yet I had neither found the urge, nor the impetus to seek divine help, until that Thursday in October. I have since paid more attention to the concept, and am as surprised as Dr. Larry Dossey, author of *Healing Words: The Power of Prayer and the Practice of Medicine*, to find evidence of a tangible benefit. Carolyn's miraculous survival of America's number one killer has certainly caused us to wonder; is it possible that prayer can heal? Trisha Meili (previously known as The Central Park Jogger) has no doubt there is a connection, and also cites Dr. Dossey's discoveries. He has uncovered scientific and medical proof that the spiritual dimension affects healing.

For instance, a cardiologist named Randolph Byrd measured prayer as a healing therapy at the Coronary Care Unit in San Francisco General Hospital. He determined that the prayed-for patients were less likely to require antibiotics, less likely to develop fluid in the lungs (called pulmonary edema, it is a common consequence of heart failure), and did not require intubation. There was also evidence of a reduced mortality, but this was not conclusive. While the research was undertaken as a scientific study and published as such, it did receive some criticism. There have been many more experiments to determine the power of spiritual, psychic and prayer-based healing. Scientists at such well-known institutions as Princeton, Harvard, and Stanford have attempted to overcome the skeptical conclusion that distant healing is mysticism. One favorable conclusion is that healing obeys laws that differ from other sciences. Another conclusion is that prayer-based healing may occur outside of conscious control. There is no doubt, however, that spiritual tools such as intercessory prayer, dreams, coincidence, and intuition have measurable, powerful, and profound effects on how we heal. And this may not be so far removed from the beliefs and practices of the witches and pagans so evident in Salem, especially in October, around the time of Halloween.

We should not ignore practices that go beyond the realm of conventional medicine, but instead consider that random or episodic events of healing have been shown, through scientific evidence, to be related and connected to a higher force at work. Dr. Dossey offers an explanation or principle for this force—he believes the mind can operate in a non-local mode. He considers that the mind is omnipresent and not limited to space and time, and at some level all minds are unitary and connected. This may explain the power of prayer, but I am not sure. I can only thank God, a few good Samaritans, the EMTs and the doctors for the miracle of Carolyn's survival.

We have always loved the change of seasons, and most especially autumn or, as I have learned to call it, the fall. I reject, however, the antediluvian preoccupation with death that pervades the month of October: Halloween and the walking dead; the death of summer; the dying leaves; and the extended darkness. I prefer to see October as a time of renewal, like it is in Australia.

Carolyn may have passed through the veil of death, but she returned, and is now protected forever—a feat not possible nor conceived by even the most powerful witches with their potions and spells. Medical technology and science has proven they are capable of overcoming the foibles of the human body. I feel that we have no need for the supernatural or superstitions of the Middle Ages. We are free to enjoy the spectacle of the "trees on fire" and the outrageous costumes without fear.

The lesson we have learned is; cherish life, and your relationships. There may be a moment when you regret not savoring the life you have now and the love you give and receive. Humans are so resilient and adaptable, that it is easy to forget how fragile we are. In seconds, your world can be altered, and you or a loved one irreversibly changed. The happiness and joy of life can be destroyed by fear, just as unconditionally as by physical trauma. A narrow escape is an opportunity to learn and grow with the knowledge. How many of us take those lessons to heart?

I do think it is a miracle that we have been given a second chance to treasure the gift of love and companionship. It could have easily slipped through our fingers.

Chapter 10

LETTING GO

Only those that risk going too far
can possibly find out how far they can go.

—T.S. Eliot

Owning an ICD is not easy. This small, shiny metal box with a complicated name is permanently installed under her skin; a hard lump in the shoulder that sets off security devices in airports and government buildings. It is a lifesaver, and cherished if it ever "goes off", but never a preferred bionic accessory. It makes life more complicated, which Carolyn sometimes finds hard to justify. Dr. Wayne Sotile describes in his book *Thriving with Heart Disease* this very issue, "The moment the device is implanted in their breasts, these men and women are beset by new physical and psychological forces they must divide and conquer." He paints a positive picture of recovery, advising that most ICD recipients adjust well, both physically and psychologically. After all, the alternative could be death.

Nevertheless retail-store doorway theft detectors are suddenly a palpable source of terror. Carolyn holds my hand tightly or insists I go through first while she grabs the back of my jacket. Sometimes I laugh off this behavior, and at other times I seek an explanation.

"What do you think will happen?" I ask, before we pass through the detector.

"*It* might go off! I'm scared."

I can see in her eyes that she doesn't really believe this. The fear so easily overcomes her rational mind, and causes her to freeze. She has not been trapped in a building the way people with phobias can be—

161

depicted so chillingly by Leonardo DiCaprio as Howard Hughes in *The Aviator*, when he cannot leave the bathroom for fear of germs on the door handle.

Carolyn and I have had many conversations about electromagnetic fields and what effect they can have on her ICD. There is an unreality about having a device inside her chest that is designed to shock her when *it* determines the need. She has been told that it is possible for the device to be "tricked" into zapping her, although the likelihood is remote. It is more likely that it will not go off as the devices have a design feature whereby strong magnetic fields disable them. It is called "magnet mode", since placing a magnet over the device results in suspension of detection and therapy, primarily for emergency suppression of the device in clinical situations. One day the manufacturers will convincingly overcome this quirk; in the meantime "retail therapy" may come with a shock beyond the price tag!

We are constantly reminded of its presence; a cuddle with my head on her chest will bring a yelp as she feels the hard metallic box rub against her rib or collarbone. It is a shame because nuzzling is one of my favorites, and now it may be permanently ruined. Carolyn even has difficulty lying on her left side, which was her favorite since she likes to sleep on the right hand side of the bed.

Buying clothes has a new twist; Carolyn now has to consider if the bump will show, among all those other devilish considerations normally accounted for in garment selection. I once joked that she might like to consider it like a breast implant—but I made that quip only the one time! I was suitably chastised, and also informed that her regular mammography scans were now an issue for her since the device is positioned just above the breast and can interfere with the scanner. Other useful medical tools are also denied her, such as MRI (Magnetic Resonance Imaging uses high-power magnetic fields to look inside the body) and even an ultrasound can be problematic. "It" will eventually be forgotten, and one day her sensitivity will recede and she will not even notice it is there. Or so they say.

Unbelievably, Carolyn had a painful reminder for many months that was neither predicted nor discussed in any detail by the medical fraternity. It was debilitating, and could have been avoided, if caught early enough. Commonly called frozen shoulder, it arises where an injury leads to lack of use due to pain. We now know that our shoulders are unstable joints because of the range of motion possible. Consequently, we have a group of muscles, tendons, and ligaments to anchor the bones in our shoulders. But problems can arise from disruption of these soft tissues as a result of injury or under-use. The medical term is capsulitis of the shoulder, and it has four distinct stages; starting with pain, then pain and stiffness, followed by stiffness and finally subsidence. Abnormal bands of tissue were growing between the joint surfaces inside Carolyn's shoulder, severely restricting her arm motion, and there may also have been a lack of synovial fluid to lubricate the joint. She only became aware of it once the shoulder was completely locked, probably because she had been favoring her left arm due to the tenderness around the wound where the ICD was implanted. And the arm sling she wore probably didn't help!

We did not know that with gentle stretching, the application of heat and non-steroidal anti-inflammatory drugs, physiotherapy could have been avoided. We also worried that if the condition deteriorated, it would be necessary for manipulation under general anesthesia, or even surgery to cut the adhesions. Carolyn was unfortunate enough to have both shoulders "freeze", one after the other, so she was most disquieted to learn from the physiotherapist that it was a common but avoidable condition. For so many months that particular legacy was a constant reminder that she had a shocking implant.

Fear, uncertainty and doubt became the hardest things for Carolyn to contend with. In my sales training we called this "FUD", and were advised to use it as a tool to persuade customers that a competitor's product or service may not be all that they claimed. In Carolyn's case, there were no competitors and no purchasing decisions to be made; her fear was self-imposed. She was terrified that her palpitations were going to cause a zap. She was uncertain when or where this might happen and doubted the device's ability to determine the difference between an arrest and her benign arrhythmia. The FUD was destabilizing her confidence just as a customer's confidence in the competitor could be shaken by that sales technique.

Carolyn was most concerned that *it* would go off while driving and she would cause an accident. She was less worried about crashing the car, but most fearful of hurting someone, even killing them. It took the mandatory six months of my chauffeuring for her to build up the confidence to drive by herself. At first she would not consider piloting the vehicle at all, especially those multilane highways where everyone seems to add twenty percent to the posted speed limit. But after a while she gained the mental fortitude to sit in the drivers seat on single lane secondary roads while I watched her carefully from the passenger seat. It is a policy, in Massachusetts, for all sudden cardiac arrest survivors to refrain from driving a car (or bus or truck for matter) for at least six months, as the statistics show that if another episode is likely, then it will occur within those twenty-six or so weeks. And of course, if it does, then driving is curtailed for another six months.

Carolyn could not accept her cardiac arrest as a real event. Perhaps it had been someone else, or it was all a dream. The device is a constant reminder, but she has no recollection of falling down or waking up in ICU. It did not happen to her. She did not see the "bright lights" or feel peaceful and "ready to go" as so many reporters of near-death expound. Carolyn has only the bump under her collarbone to verify the event. Did it really happen? She could confer with the three managers in her office if the deception became too palpable. They had witnessed the event and could verify the reality for her. But even that was not enough to defy her denial. Meeting Tom and Sara again made a huge dent in her armor of denial; the tears in their eyes revealed all as they held her in a warm embrace. Carolyn felt it was almost spiritual. She began to accept her unknown experience after that reunion.

And it was a reunion in many ways. When Carolyn returned to Dallas to complete the management course eight months later, she had the same instructors, in the same hotel, and gave the same morning introduction. As you can imagine, she felt highly stressed and was praised for her fortitude. It was a form of therapy, facing the demons, but also an attempt to evoke some memories.

But when the arrhythmia returned she did not feel so brave.

"I was a sitting duck for it, and felt so nervous that the palpitations were non-stop," she said later, fully expecting to have had another episode, almost forgetting she was protected this time.

෯

I believe Carolyn's biggest challenge was accepting the significance of the statement "pupils fixed and dilated" written on her admitting chart. She felt uneasy that another term "clinically dead" also applied. Carolyn's electrophysiologist in Boston explained to us that the term fixed and dilated indicates that the brain stem is cut off, or not functioning, which he said is not the same as death, "but is certainly not good". He also confided in us that it is rare for arrest victims to survive, but in his opinion "…that is your story all over. She shouldn't be here." He had a further comment for Carolyn that stuck in our minds. "Your body requires very little to keep going. However, without the ICD, next time you won't be here."

෯

As I have said before, Carolyn is a fighter, to which I attribute her survival after she reached the ER. She would not let sudden cardiac arrest triumph over her, and strives to regain her life unaffected by the event. Not surprisingly, Carolyn has maintained her working life, even increasing her achievements and status within the company. She has some degree of celebrity within the organization, but usually keeps the episode private, unless she meets one of the few hundred managers present that Thursday in October, or the issue of AED deployment and EMS response times arises. She has found several other "bionic" women in the company and marvels at the coincidence in their gender and age group. Not being alone in having an ICD has helped her realize there is no stigma or blemish associated with it. In fact, she is better off than the rest of us, since we are the ones who are unprotected now.

Trisha Meili wrote that the decision to announce her identity as the Central Park Jogger represented an important breakthrough in her healing. Her resolve to reveal the details of her rehabilitation impressed me, both as a therapeutic measure for herself and other head trauma victims and to prove that a life need not be destroyed so easily. She also wrote that coming so close to death must transform a person in some way. That story reminded me that, while Carolyn's physical healing was complete, she would require many months, if not years, to adjust to the fact that it occurred at all. I agree that a close encounter with death certainly transforms the survivor and that it doesn't always mean a loss; positive changes are possible.

At one stage Carolyn wondered what message her arrest might signify. She considered that the V-fib might have been a warning from her body to say "enjoy your life and fully experience the physical or I'll stop," perhaps informing her that if you don't appreciate your body it withers away and dies. The reasoning didn't last long on inspection, but the concept certainly took hold. Both our lives are richer and better than before, and we cherish the second chance she has been given. We are committed to helping others affected by sudden cardiac arrest as a means to recuperation, physiologically if not spiritually. We have attended local ICD support groups and enjoyed their meetings where we could assist new members to this exclusive club. Many of them were not sure they are so lucky to belong, but we know that's just a passing phase, and that the alternative is to not belong to anything ever again.

In my research on how and why this occurred to Carolyn, I came across other instances of catastrophic medical problems arising spontaneously, or from obscure or unknown causes. Robert McCrum fought the terrible affects of an idiopathic medical emergency—in his case a stroke—to regain his publishing life. He chronicled the recovery in a memoir, *My Year Off*, and in particular, points out the difficulty with how suddenly his life had changed. He had to make changes in lifestyle, but did he not let the fragility of a circulatory infarct destroy his life.

I am particularly touched by the coincidences between our stories, although the genders are reversed and the medical complaint was different. At the age of forty-two, he had been married to his American wife, Sarah, only a few months earlier, and they were separated by a great distance due to a business trip when his spouse was informed of the devastating news. She, too, had the dread and fear to accompany her on the long airplane flight, as I had, with little or no reliable information on the cause or cure. She, too, had sat by his side in ICU, with his life in the balance, patiently waiting for him to come alive. In a disturbing way it was comforting to read that they also had a harrowing time with the neurologists. Sarah was particularly concerned about the effects of the trauma—that "severe insult to the brain"—and with good reason, as he had suffered considerable damage. Carolyn and I feel favored to be spared the horrible repercussions of oxygen deprived brain cells.

Robert says he's not troubled by the knowledge that there was no treatment that would have prevented his stroke, or even an explanation as to why it occurred, despite the conclusive pathology describing what had had happened to his brain. I cannot say that Carolyn or I are as accepting or comfortable with the lack of explanation for her sudden cardiac arrest. Maybe as a journalist McCrum is more able to accept things as they are. Or is he just wiser?

♀

A major barrier to releasing the fear and intrusion that ICD ownership provokes is the regular checkup. As with all emergency life saving equipment, an ICD must be tested to ensure it is operating correctly. The test requires regularly reliving the cardiac arrest episode, for the life of the device. As is the way with most professions, there is an acronym for the test. It is called a NIPS, or Non Invasive Programmed Stimulation.

Just as it did in Dallas, this procedure remains the most frightening time of our lives. Nothing can adequately prepare us. Her precious heart has to be stilled. An electric shock does the job. Only a small shock, but it is delivered at just the right time and in exactly the right place. She will have no pulse, and thus no life giving oxygen for her brain and organs. Her blood pressure and heart rhythm are monitored to ensure the precise conditions are achieved. But she is sedated so she does not feel any pain, or suffer in any way. And she is almost guaranteed to survive.

We can never forget.

The NIPS test is designed to check the ICD battery and electrical connections to ensure the device will work when needed. It is called non-invasive as there is no surgery involved (i.e. the skin is not cut), but it is certainly a serious hospital based procedure, involving a general anesthetic and defibrillation. Usually, the test is performed in a specialty care area, either an electrophysiology lab or a catheterization lab, where a wand, looking suspiciously like a computer mouse, is placed on the patient's chest to communicate with the device through the skin by magnetism. The medical technician commands the device to "induce" an abnormal rhythm and then monitors how well the device treats the arrhythmia. It is policy for the manufacturer's representative to be present at a NIPS test to assist with any complications or configuration issues with the device. Precise electrical and timing measurements are taken to assess the generator, leads and the efficacy of the ICD system. The evaluation also requires a blood test and an electrocardiogram (EKG). Blood pressure, pulse and oxygen levels are monitored throughout the procedure. It is possible that the abnormal rhythm will be induced multiple times to insure proper treatment or modification to the programmable settings in the device. Of course, the abnormal rhythm is corrected by the device automatically, and usually consumes two weeks worth of battery power each time. So Carolyn is guaranteed to have the device zap her every few years. At least she will know about it in advance.

Once discharged from a NIPS, a responsible adult is required to take the patient home, as they are unable to drive for twenty-four hours. It is not a trivial appointment and usually reveals some disturbing trends in the patient's cardiac activity, for the device keeps a record of all abnormal heart rhythms. This data is downloaded during the test and analyzed by the electrophysiologist.

After less than a dozen of these non-invasive tests it will be time for a positively invasive procedure, the removal of the device. Depending upon usage and battery strength, the device will need to be replaced at least every decade. An ICD's microprocessor, capacitor and battery are hermitically sealed inside a titanium shell, and once the battery is exhausted the whole unit is renewed. Apparently there is a benefit to this foible; each generation of device has been smaller, more powerful and longer lasting than the previous one. Carolyn was given a fourth generation unit, (the same model that Vice President Dick Cheney had installed the year before) and has small consolation that one day she will receive a future generation device that could well be unnoticeable and miniaturized like so many semiconductor devices have become.

Letting go certainly entails accepting that the machine is going to zap her, and that it is a wondrous thing if it does. The alternative is not living at all, but we hope that the day the device will be appreciated doesn't come.

༄

Part of the process of letting go is to recognize the ramifications and effects of the calamity, and just accept them. I was touched by the reaction and actions of Carolyn's colleagues. Not only did her boss, Jim, display familial care and concern, but Sara, the manager in charge of the course, reached out to all attendees to thank them and help them feel at ease—to lessen the fright and deal with the shock. I have included the email Sara sent to all the staff that witnessed Carolyn's collapse, since her words were so poignant.

Sara Smith/Fort Worth/IBM   10/13/2002 05:52 PM
Subject   A reflection as we begin again on Monday

Dear ones,
I wanted to get a note to you all as we take a deep breath and begin
our work lives once more tomorrow. I wanted to thank you for the
place you will always have in my life. You are to me the embodiment
of great courage, great faith and great hope from those who used
your skills to save Carolyn's life in those precious moments, to the
others who bathed those working in prayer. Collectively you did what
it took: you made telephone calls, you found health care workers,
you held each other, you went to the hospital, you stepped into
leadership, you stood back and let leadership emerge, and you
stayed at the hotel to continue our work. All of those acts took
courage, faith and hope. And all were important.
In a moment we became united in something so much larger than
numbers and sales and quarters. Despite everything, you chose to
stay and the work you did in Dallas reflected your enormous affection
and respect for each other. It is my wish for you to take all those
experiences and know that we were at our very best the best we
could be in all those moments.
Tomorrow calls us all back and much of the world won't know how
much we've changed. But we will. Feel free to look at those around
you differently. Prioritize your activities differently. Live your lives
newly. Take care of yourselves, my friends. You are precious.

Regards, Sara C. Smith
Sales Transformation Manager
Professional Co-Active Coach
IBM Sales Transformation Management Team

Letting go is a hard thing to do. Accepting change, forgiving and not
being afraid to move on, leaving behind the old and taking the lessons
to heart. These emotional wrestling matches we often tackle in the
background and almost unconsciously. But after a momentous event
these issues become important and urgent. Carolyn is now aware of the
stress she creates for herself, both at work and at home. The change at
home was easy—she now appreciates our glorious life every day and
will not allow anything to impinge upon it. She blames me for the
wonderful daily lifestyle we enjoy, but I know she has changed inside.
Carolyn has a new perspective, one that is less brittle and controlling,

and is now more accepting and flexible. Work, however, is another realm and harder to insulate, especially when others make careless or ill considered decisions. Situations that invoke high emotion in the office, those seemingly important issues, now appear a little ridiculous and trivial. Carolyn has decided to tackle only those valuable and gratifying opportunities: the things that matter to her. Those that are not so important don't need to be fought. Fortuitously, she is being rewarded with each step, recognized by superiors who also value the bigger picture.

∾

Confronting death is, well, confronting. Carolyn continues to wonder at the miracle of her survival, but is no longer afraid. She is free of the "burden of living"; she once felt a duty to stay alive. Her reanimation has given her a gift—the realization that she is mortal and only here for the merest instant. So she now makes the most of each day, cherishing the moments of happiness and delight, and leaving behind the discontent and defeats. Maybe the motto should be, "Disappointment never makes for a happy past, and is the product of our attitudes anyway".

Carolyn told me, in that delicious matter of fact manner of hers, "It is the people left behind that matter in a person's demise. They have so much to deal with, but I will be gone."

∾

I, too, have had to adjust. I did not want my wife to die. It had been a delight to watch her bloom, revealing the goodness I had seen that wonderful evening we first met in Sydney. Just as a cicada sheds its crinkly scales, giving rise to a fresh new beauty, I relished seeing her shed that protective scaly veneer, toughened by emotional hardship and twenty years of harsh Australian sun, to emerge renewed and alive with enthusiasm and wonder at the joy of love. It appeared as though the real Carolyn was waking up, seeing the world through new eyes that revealed the wonders and gifts before us. Like a child growing up, she was constantly having "firsts", and experiencing the excitement that brings. I felt a paternal instinct warming the cold heart of my self-centered, only-child form of selfishness. I am grateful to have learned to value the time we have together, and make it special whenever given the chance.

Some believe in fate, but I believe that *I* am responsible for making my life the way it is. Carolyn's sudden cardiac arrest was not part of the plan and I could not control it. Nor could she. Luckily, she survived, since I am not sure I could have continued without her.

Carolyn has given me more than all of my previous romantic entanglements. I am a firm believer in the principle that love is a selfish act, and I am a selfish person. Carolyn's ecstasy is my motive and justification. I do not spoil her, but she gets more than she thinks she deserves. In return, I get everything I could possibly want, and we prosper together.

Each morning she wakes up, looks at me, asks for a "special cuddle", and says, "I'm so lucky, because you adore me," to which I reply, "*I'm* the lucky one."

EPILOGUE

What does not kill me makes me stronger.
                              –Johann Wolfgang von Goethe

Carolyn passed the one-thousand-day anniversary without being zapped, and hopefully she never will receive that surprise "kick in the chest". I sometimes think she would be calmer and less fearful of the device if it actually did go off. We have had conversations with other owners who have had "events" and they do admit that the apprehension dissolves after that first time. However, I did notice that, in its place, they had some anxiety that it may go off again!

Living with an ICD is still not so easy.

We have not allowed that episode in Dallas to alter our lives. If any change has occurred it is for the better. We appreciate the moments, especially those selfish times when we are alone, but together. There is tenderness and possessiveness in the way we interact now. Where we thought we were invincible, we now realize we are adaptable. When issues arise we are quick to see the pitfall of harboring resentment or regrets. Carolyn has an arrhythmia that was benign, although it became malignant that one time. Now, she is protected against its deadly consequences. She has a device, which needs to be tested regularly. Consequently, each time we move house there is a new relationship to be made, for the device cannot "survive" without a special type of cardiologist—an electrophysiologist. There is a hard lump in Carolyn's chest, and I must be gentle on that side. She also has a scar, but you would have to know it was there to see it. She occasionally complains about the bump, but accepts that it will be smaller when the device is replaced, probably many times in the future.

We are both grateful she has "clean pipes", and that Randy and Tom were so quick to act. We have let go the demons, and are committed to helping others learn what sudden cardiac arrest is, and what can be done to avoid the devastation it wreaks if ignored.

∾

Too often sudden cardiac death strikes down people whose hearts are not ready, but they can be saved. Claude Beck, a professor of surgery in Cleveland coined the phrase "hearts too good to die" in 1947 when developing the then emerging defibrillator programs. He felt that sudden cardiac arrest was taking otherwise healthy and valuable lives unnecessarily, and vowed to stop the carnage. I was so taken by his perspective when researching sudden cardiac arrest, both for my own education, and also for material for this book, that I felt it was the perfect title. Not only was Carolyn's heart muscle not ready, but also her spirit was indomitable. In my eyes, she truly is too good to die.

I do accept that without the intervention of a defibrillator, Carolyn would not have lived. It is a credit to those pioneers and the Minnesota "medical alley" manufacturers that we have such technology. In Claude's era the large heavy devices were wheeled up to the patient, but now they are as light and transportable as a laptop computer. In his day they were strictly manual machines, requiring expert training, whereas now the portable devices are fully automatic, and have been given the acronym AED, which stands for Automatic External Defibrillator. The technology has improved enormously in the last two decades, so much so that the special internal defibrillators—always called ICDs—have been made so small and light that they can be surgically implanted during a relatively simple operation that takes only a few hours. The earlier units required open-heart surgery and were not long-lived devices. Unfortunately, that implied their owners were also not long lived.

∾

I wrote this book for Carolyn's benefit as much as yours. She missed nearly everything we went through, and yet for most of it she was

174

there. Maybe you have some memories and experiences missing too? I decided to write a book of our adventure since, when I sought to understand the fear and shock we endured, I was able to find much of that emotion expressed in written form. So did Carolyn—from the same book! It was *An Arrow Through The Heart*, by Deborah Daw Heffernan, The Free Press, 2002.

Since then, we have both read widely on the subject, and participated in survivor advocacy events. The likelihood of surviving a sudden cardiac arrest is so remote that the impact of speaking with a survivor is potent. The pair of us have been active on the national level with both the American Heart Association (AHA) and National Centre for Early Defibrillation (NCED), lobbying Congress. We had a full day of meetings to persuade each of the federal members from Massachusetts; Senator Edward Kennedy, Senator John Kerry, Rep. Marty Meehan, and Rep. Edward Markey, that the country needs continued, sustained investment in medical research. It was exciting and enlightening to visit those senators and representatives in their offices, and show them the true value of their legislative decisions. The personal story of a constituent has a powerful effect on a politician. We feel some responsibility for the decision to expand Medicare coverage for ICDs, and increase the budget allocation for the National Institutes of Health (NIH) funding of heart and stroke research in 2005.

When sudden cardiac arrest affects your life or someone close to you, it is often difficult to deal with the issues. I recommend you find a support group to share your story and emotions. The hospital, or your electrophysiologist is sure to offer an education and support network for patients and their families to deal with the concerns and answer questions. The meetings are informal and are often attended by a physician who will cover the important topics troubling you and your family. This provides the chance to express your thoughts and feelings to caring, knowledgeable professionals outside of the clinical environment. We have both found that listening to other survivors has helped in the mental adjustment and acceptance of the device.

At one memorable ICD support group meeting, we were impressed by a wonderfully active and sprightly lady who had decided to call the device her "titanium jewelry"!

Unfortunately, sudden cardiac arrest is not likely to be cured in the foreseeable future, so there will be many more spouses and friends that will want to know what happened and why. Some will find a reason, others will not. The medical technology and terminology can be difficult to understand, let alone remember, but that is only part of knowing. It can be difficult to accept what happened. We find that the days can go by without a reminder, but usually within a week there will be a trigger and the emotions bubble up again.

༈

I believe that liberation and self-determination can come from letting go of fear. And I have found that knowledge can give me the power to let go. If I can learn about something before I have to experience it, I am far less anxious, and thus more able to perform and prevail. For that reason I have included some complex and technical medical material in a separate chapter. I do not profess to be an expert, nor qualified in medicine, but much of this information is freely available, and often discussed between patients and their specialists. I think it valuable to share my learning with you; maybe it will entice you to do your own research. I am often reminded that one's learning can translate from a previous experience to new ones.

You may not like to read the long paragraphs of detailed technical material, but I have often found them helpful in dispelling the unknown—probably a result of my engineering background. In my case, understanding the technicalities was important so that I could appreciate what the physicians were telling us (or *not* telling us). Often the complexity overwhelmed me, but some of it stuck. I have put some of the facts and figures at the end of the story for this purpose, and you can decide if they are important to you or not.

WHAT CAN WE DO TO STOP THEM DYING?

A single death is a tragedy; a million deaths is a statistic.

—Joseph Stalin

Cardiac emergencies often have the highest fatality rates simply because they demand the fastest response times. During a sudden cardiac arrest, every minute that passes without an appropriate emergency response translates into an eight to ten percent reduction in the chance of survival. Many people have learned the value of automated external defibrillators (AEDs) in saving lives, which has been callously described; "If there's been no CPR and no defibrillation, you might as well send the hearse."

Over ninety percent of sudden cardiac arrest victims die because they didn't have quick access to this easy-to-administer lifesaving treatment. By making more people aware of sudden cardiac arrest, and by improving access to AEDs, we can increase the survival rate. We can create a HeartSafe Community by linking the levels of emergency cardiac care, and creating the "Chain of Survival". Several organizations are expert in this field and provide public assistance and training. On a national level there is the American Heart Association and the Red Cross, and specifically focused on cardiac arrest is the Sudden Cardiac Arrest Association SCAA (previously National Center for Early Defibrillation NCED) and the Sudden Cardiac Arrest Foundation.

The fight to save them began a long time ago. The origins of the procedures and principles so conscientiously employed today began before either Australia or America was classed as a nation, but late in the twentieth century it all came together.

The quest for a solution to sudden death spans two centuries, from the English rescue societies of the 1770s, to the early 1970s when three critical components were put in place: cardiopulmonary resuscitation, defibrillation and swift pre-hospital care. We no longer have to accept sudden death as inevitable, unlike the ancient Celts, the physicians of the Middle Ages, or the medical schools of the 1950s. There is still a long way to go to help the millions of souls lost each year to sudden cardiac death around the world. The journey has just begun, and while today death from heart problems is not absolute, the road is littered with insight, or should I say hindsight?

One hundred years ago, heart disease was a killer; you were old and you died. Forty years ago we learned that smoking kills. (You may not know that World War II created more deaths *after* the war than during it—from the addicts to all those free smokes handed out!) Thirty years ago, cholesterol research uncovered that (now) widely known risk indicator. Twenty years ago stroke was identified as a killer, (while not strictly a heart problem, stroke is often caused by an arterial blockage and is thus related to circulation). Only ten years ago, AEDs were useful lifesavers but deemed too expensive and dangerous for widespread use. Today, they can be purchased over the counter for around the cost of a high definition television. And most recently, Medicare approved reimbursement of ICDs for nearly eighty percent of the highest risk patients.

৵

Hundreds of thousands of Americans die each year of a cardiac arrest within one hour of the onset of symptoms, and *before* they reach the hospital. But if CPR was administered immediately, and an AED was deployed within five minutes, over two hundred people per day would still be alive, and it could very well be someone you know.

There are two fundamental prerequisites, CPR and AEDs, which fortify "The Chain of Survival".

Cardiopulmonary resuscitation (literally heart lung resuscitation) is a relatively recent life saving procedure, although, it does have origins as far back as the 16th century. The three elements to resuscitation are: a clear airway, respiration and circulation. They can be simply remembered as the ABCs—Airway, Breathing and Circulation. It was not until the early 1960s that this was clearly understood and defined as a procedure. Peter Safar is one of those credited with developing CPR, documenting his findings in 1957, and later presenting them to the Maryland Medical Society in 1960. The US Army also assisted in the widespread adoption of the once controversial mouth-to-mouth technique. In 1958 the American Medical Association (AMA) endorsed this "expired air breathing" practice in favor of the accepted manual methods, many of which involved lifting the patients' arms and pressing on their ribcage to inflate and deflate the lungs. But it was not until 1962 that the American Heart Association (AHA) proposed the term cardiopulmonary resuscitation.

Nearly two centuries earlier, in 1767, the Society for Recovery of Drowned Persons was established in Amsterdam. This group was the first to initiate a concerted, organized effort to deal with sudden and unexpected deaths. A wave of such societies was soon created throughout Europe. This was remarkable because not many years prior it was considered sacrilegious to interfere with those recently dead. Bringing back the dead was not a function that mere mortals should perform.

After the "Enlightenment" of the 18th century, death was no longer passively accepted. The search for the properties of life had begun in earnest, although, at that time, little was known about circulation and respiration. Restoring the life force, or reanimation as it was called, was clumsy and crude, not to mention unreliable. It was common for resuscitation to take six or more hours, with treatments such as tickling, blowing tobacco smoke into the mouth or rectum, and bloodletting. Thank goodness medical knowledge has progressed since that time!

The standards for CPR in the United States were established, and are regularly updated by the American Heart Association. More than six million people each year receive CPR training from instructors taught by the AHA. Often, local fire departments conduct free CPR training sessions for their neighborhoods because they intimately know the value of early bystander CPR. As a result of these efforts, one in two sudden cardiac arrest victims receive CPR before the emergency services arrive. Performing CPR early can double the likelihood of survival. Do you know how to do it? Would you be prepared to help a stranger?

❧

Although there is a report as far back as 1774 in London, of the electrical stimulus of an apparently dead child, defibrillation as a technique for resuscitation was first postulated in the late-nineteenth-century. There were growing concerns over unexpected sudden deaths due to the increasing use of chloroform anesthesia and the incidence of accidental electrocution.

Carolyn's savior may actually be Claude Beck, the professor of surgery at Western Reserve University in Cleveland, who developed a defibrillator for use directly on the heart muscle. He based his design on the work of an electrical engineer, William Kouwenhoven, and a medical doctor, Donald Hooker, who had undertaken research in the 1930s on behalf of the Rockefeller Institute and Consolidated Electric Company, to help deal with fatal accidents involving electricity. Dr. Beck realized that ventricular fibrillation often occurred in hearts that were otherwise sound, and coined the phrase "hearts too good to die". His electric shock procedure required open-heart surgery, but did save lives as early as 1947. It took a Bostonian, Dr. Paul Zoll, to develop the external defibrillator, which he had manufactured in Massachusetts by Electrodyne. This "miracle" device could accomplish "complete recovery ...without ill effect to the patient", and was written up in the *New England Journal of Medicine* in 1956. Both the Beck and Zoll defibrillators were large, heavy instruments that required mains electric alternating current (AC). Another doctor, Bernard Lown from Johns Hopkins, solved the portability issue, when he discovered that direct current (DC) was just as effective, as well as being safer and easier to generate from batteries. The first use of his newly developed DC device was at Peter Bent Brigham Hospital in Boston in 1961. Before long, portable defibrillators were widely available, and manufactured by several companies.

Unlike those early defibrillators, the current AED units automatically determine if a shock is required, and autonomously select and deliver the appropriate energy level. They are easy to use and safe for untrained bystanders to operate, as the user cannot override a "no shock" advisory by the AED, thus protecting the patient.

Despite the fact that AEDs are not as ubiquitous as a fire extinguisher—omnipresent and ready in case of emergency—they *are* regularly used throughout the country, saving lives nearly every day. Late one April evening in 2004, a lucky fellow was revived using an AED at a Boston transit train station. He was lucky because the inspector on the platform had been trained in using an AED only eight months earlier, and it was one of only six stations that had a device. Unfortunately, there was not the same emergency care available two years earlier, in 2002, when a 61-year-old scientist with the U.S. Geological Survey collapsed on board a similar train. He was pronounced dead on arrival at the hospital. The train authority has decided to deploy dozens more of these devices at train and bus stops throughout Boston.

All AEDs approved for use in the United States are designed to be used by non-medical operators, and utilize a synthesized voice to prompt users through each step. This ease of use has given rise to the notion of public access defibrillation (PAD) programs, which could well be the greatest advance in the treatment of out-of-hospital cardiac arrest.

While the deployment of defibrillators is becoming more widespread, they are not as prevalent as they ought to be. It has been suggested that only one in two ambulances, less than fifteen percent of first-response fire department vehicles, and less than one percent of police vehicles carry defibrillators. (Page, Richard L. Et al, *Use of Automated External Defibrillators by a U.S. Airline, New England Journal of Medicine*, October 26, 2000.)

Widespread deployment of defibrillators within your community could decrease the collapse-to-shock time and improve the survival rates. A study published in the *New England Journal of Medicine* indicated that survival rates are highest when defibrillation is delivered within three minutes of the time of collapse. Although there is no formula for determining the optimal number of defibrillators and their placement, it is best to install the devices in locations where large numbers of people gather, such as offices, sports fields, transport hubs, retail stores and malls. Look around where you live, where you work, and the places you frequent and determine how close you are to a defibrillator. If a potential victim can't be reached within the three to five minute window, it may be time to become a champion for early defibrillation. Not just for your safety, but for others as well.

The American Heart Association developed the "Chain of Survival" concept in 1990, and evokes the emergency medical services continuum pioneered by Peter Safar, who coined the term "life support chain". The Chain of Survival specifies a series of critical steps that can help save lives during cardiovascular emergencies, and although specifically designed for sudden cardiac arrest, all unresponsive victims can benefit from activating the Chain. It is a four-step intervention process that should be implemented quickly and efficiently. Each of the steps must be put into motion within the first few minutes of a cardiac arrest, starting with *Early Access*—Call 9-1-1 and get an AED. The next step is *Early CPR*—"Pump and Blow" which should be started and maintained until the first responders arrive. Third step is *Early Defibrillation*—Use the AED! If one is available it should be used, as an AED is the only thing that can re-start the heart function of a person with ventricular fibrillation. And the final step is *Early Advanced Care*—EMS. Administered by paramedics and other highly trained EMS personnel, cardiac drugs and breathing tubes can help sustain a normal rhythm after successful defibrillation.

Early access is easiest to achieve with 9-1-1 systems and widespread community education and publicity. In 1999, 190 million calls were placed to 9-1-1, and 50 million of those were made from cell phones. The number of calls to 9-1-1 from mobile phone users is rising dramatically each year, highlighting the importance of early access and this should be reinforced during CPR classes. Early CPR helps patients by slowing the process of dying, but its effectiveness diminishes within minutes. Early recognition and early CPR are best achieved when the community is well informed about cardiac emergencies and well trained in CPR. The earliest possible delivery of defibrillation is critical, and by itself can be sufficient to save victims of sudden cardiac death. (American Heart Association; *Chain of Survival Fact Sheet.*)

Without the quick response of Tom and Randy, it is unlikely that Carolyn would have survived her arrest, and at best she would have sustained neurological damage. If the EMTs did not have an AED on-board, Carolyn would certainly have died. If the hotel she was attending had an AED on-site, the danger would have been reduced immensely. That particular hotel has had two instances of sudden cardiac arrest—the other victim died. Now that Carolyn has an ICD, she is protected all day, every day, but we did not know she required one until she suffered that terrifying collapse.

There are many causes of that chaotic and deadly rhythm which kills so efficiently, but sometimes the reasons elude us. Carolyn's case is of interest to nearly every electrophysiologist we meet, and they all accept that it was idiopathic. It is a specialist field, and I do not pretend to be an authority, however, I would like to share with you some causes of sudden cardiac arrest that I found interesting.

The Brugada syndrome, a hereditary disease named after the three Spanish-born physician brothers who investigated the disorder, is a form of sudden cardiac death prevalent in young adults. The first discovery in 1986, of the disease by Dr. Pedro Brugada indicated that genetic abnormalities were linked to the syndrome, and pointed to it being a disease affecting the cardiac electrical system. And, Dr. Ramon Brugada, Jr., a molecular cardiologist from Baylor College of Medicine, was instrumental in determining the genetic basis and molecular mechanism for idiopathic ventricular fibrillation.

A parent with the Brugada syndrome usually has a fifty-percent chance of transmitting the disease to his/her offspring. It is believed to account for nearly five percent of cases of sudden cardiac death worldwide. In some regions of Southeast Asia, it is the second most common reason for death for men under the age of forty. (Death from car accidents is more common!) In northern Thailand, it is the leading natural cause of death in young men, and is known as Lai Tai (death during sleep). According to local superstition, widow ghosts come to take them away in their sleep, prompting many young men to go to bed at night dressed as women, with the hope they could fool the ghost. In the Philippines, the phenomenon is known as Bangungut (scream followed by sudden death during sleep), and in Japan it is called Pokkuri (unexpected sudden death at night). Others call it SUDS, or Sudden Unexpected Death Syndrome. It has been suggested that Australian medical practitioners need to be aware of this condition, as it is particularly relevant in my home country, where approximately half-a-million of the population were born in Southeast Asia. Treatment for the syndrome includes implantation of an ICD.

Similar to Brugada, long QT syndrome (or LQTS) is an inherited condition and involves a disturbance to the heart's electrical system. It affects the recharging of the electrical system after each heartbeat and is caused by dysfunction of the ion channels. These channels control the flow of potassium, sodium and calcium ions across the cell membrane. The flow of these ions in and out of the cells produces the electrical activity of the heart. One form of LQTS, called Romano-Ward Syndrome, appears in twice as many females as males.

The QT interval is a measure of the time required for depolarization and repolarization of heart cells. Mutations of at least six genes have been identified as the cause of a congenital long QT syndrome that renders patients vulnerable to a very fast, abnormal heart rhythm known as torsade de pointes. Sudden loss of consciousness during physical exertion or high emotion can be an indicator of long QT syndrome. One in three people with the syndrome never exhibit symptoms and are usually only diagnosed by an electrocardiogram. Fortunately, beta-blocker medications are an effective long-term therapy for most patients, and short-term treatment with potassium and magnesium is also helpful. But of course, an ICD is recommended for those less fortunate.

❧

I was stunned to find out that everyone's heart is vulnerable to electrical disturbance when relaxing from a ventricular contraction. It is incredible that all of us are susceptible to V-fib at this particularly sensitive point in the heart rhythm, which is called the T-wave.

While Carolyn's sudden cardiac arrest was deemed idiopathic, it is generally accepted that she was the victim of a premature ventricular contraction (PVC) at a critical point in the repolarization of her heart muscle cells. This delicate cycle of chemical and electrical conditions, called the action potential, is essential to proper functioning of the myocardial cells, the workhorse of the heart muscle. The ion channels mentioned earlier are the source of the electrical currents that cause the myocardial cells to contract, and if disrupted they can affect the responsiveness of the cells, and thus affect the heart rhythm. Medications such as beta-blockers are designed to act upon these same ion channels to control a patient's heart functions.

PVCs are often due to premature depolarization of the myocardial cells, and are not particularly dangerous unless they occur in pairs, triplets, or more than three beats in a row. In that situation, there is a danger that the unstable chemical and electrical status will cause changes in the membrane channel that leads to electrophysiologic dysfunction. This may cause automatic activity or reentrant circuits that will escalate into V-tach or V-fib, with lethal consequences.

Despite the idiopathic term implying a lack of understanding or definitive knowledge, one aspect is well established: non-uniform cardiac recovery properties reduce the threshold for V-fib, increasing the likelihood of a sudden cardiac arrest. I urge you to consider this medical mayhem as a background to understanding the forces at work inside our bodies, and the miracle of our persistence within such a fragile system.

✦

Regardless of the cause, sudden cardiac arrest is deadly. Luckily, there is a powerful countermeasure available to us. Following on from CPR training and AED deployment is a community program supported by the American Heart Association, and sponsored by many state governments. It is called the HeartSafe Community Program, and encourages communities to strengthen the Chain of Survival by awarding points, called "heartbeats", to cities and towns that achieve specific targets in the number of residents with CPR training and the number of first responder vehicles equipped with AEDs. Residents and visitors will know when they have entered a HeartSafe Community by road signage denoting the city or town's HeartSafe status.

PUBLIC ACCESS DEFIBRILLATION (PAD) PROGRAMS

There is something fascinating about science.
One gets such wholesale returns of conjecture
out of such a trifling investment of fact.

–Mark Twain

Public access to defibrillation is the term given to the action of non-medical persons who respond to out-of-hospital cardiac arrests. It involves delivering the technology of defibrillation and associated training to the community. The American Heart Association Board of Directors approved support of this program in June 1995. One of the key aspects of a PAD program is making Automatic External Defibrillators available in public or private places where large numbers of people gather, and where people who are at high risk for heart attacks reside.`

AEDs have revolutionized out of hospital defibrillation because they have eliminated the need for rhythm-recognition training. AEDs identify ventricular fibrillation more rapidly than manual defibrillation techniques and require less time to achieve defibrillation. Their use has resulted in increased survival rates and improved prognoses for patients in cardiac arrest.

New York State has mandated AEDs be provided for all schools and athletic events. Illinois passed a similar law. In California, they want to make defibrillators as common as fire extinguishers. The Philadelphia School District estimates that as many as seven thousand American children and youths die annually from SCA, and have equipped their school gyms and playing fields with AEDs to fight this devastation.

In 1993, only fourteen percent of arrest victims were saved in Boston. Mayor Menino was determined to improve that rate and make Boston's EMS among the nation's best. It took a decade, and in 2004, Boston saved forty percent of cardiac arrest victims. Of all the nation's biggest cities, Seattle was the safest with a forty five percent survival rate. Early access to defibrillation is a major factor in achieving these dramatic improvements.

Many businesses have taken the initiative to invest in AEDs rather than expose themselves to the types of lawsuits that were initiated shortly after the introduction of the fire extinguisher. An AED is similar in size and cost to a laptop computer, and one day might be as prevalent.

GOOD SAMARITAN LAWS

All fifty U.S. states have Good Samaritan laws, giving some immunity to laypeople that help others in distress. These laws specifically grant immunity to volunteers who assist strangers in emergency situations, including using an AED on another person. The laws vary from state to state, but generally limit or eliminate the liability of a volunteer rescuer.

On the federal level, President Clinton signed the Cardiac Arrest Survival Act (CASA) into law on November 13, 2000, as part of the Public Health Improvement Act. (In May of that same year, a visitor to the White House collapsed and was revived using an AED). The act requires the U.S. Secretary of Health and Human Services to establish guidelines for placing AEDs in federal buildings, and protects users, purchasers and trainers from litigation following emergency use of an AED. An important provision of the CASA act provides AED users with conditional Good Samaritan legal liability immunity for any harm resulting from the use or attempted use of the device. One of its primary goals is to encourage people to respond in a cardiac emergency by using an AED.

Congress also passed The Rural Access to Emergency Devices Act (also called the Rural AED Act) along with the CASA Act. This law authorizes the appropriation of $25 million in grants to certain "community partnerships" for the purchase of AEDs and training.

In all Canadian provinces, volunteer rescuers who use AEDs in an emergency have liability protection.

The Airline Passenger Safety Act, enacted in April 1998, requires the Federal Aviation Administration (FAA) to review the contents of medical kits carried on commercial airplanes. Administrative rules proposed by the FAA, as required by this law, mandate that every commercial aircraft be equipped with specified life-saving equipment and appropriately stocked first-aid and medical kits, including AEDs, and that flight crew members be trained in their use.

AED LEGISLATION

Unfortunately, State laws and regulations are not uniform. Some states do not oversee the use of AEDs, and the scope of oversight varies widely in those that do. The legislation affecting early defibrillation programs address two key elements; individuals specifically permitted to use AEDs, known as "user classes", and litigation. User classes include; emergency medical responders, such as paramedics and emergency medical technicians; public safety emergency responders, such as firefighters and police officers; targeted emergency responders, such as security guards, industrial first-aid staff, flight attendants, ship crews, ski patrol, lifeguards, non-hospital healthcare facility workers, nursing home personnel, retirement community personnel, athletic trainers, and others. In addition, the classes include trained citizen responders, such as friends, relatives and co-workers of people with identified heart problems.

Successful litigation against an AED user requires four essential legal elements. These include duty, breach of duty, causation of injury, and legally recognized damages. A negligence claim cannot succeed if *any one* of these elements is missing. Since a bystander has no legal obligation to provide medical aid to an ill or injured person, even if the bystander has the ability to help, breach of duty cannot be proven.

189

HOTELS

Carlson Hotels Worldwide announced in 2003 that it had installed AEDs in twenty-one U.S. properties. The Regent International Hotels, Radisson Hotels & Resorts and Country Inns & Suites By Carlson were the first to have a strategy to install LIFEPAK® CR Plus AEDs in all of their owned and managed U.S. hotels.

The Disney Company has deployed more than one hundred AEDs at Disneyland®, their flagship theme park in Anaheim, California. Venues such as Marriott, Knott's Berry Farm and Harrah's Casinos have placed AEDs in conspicuous locations to let people know they're safe from sudden cardiac arrest while visiting the establishments.

In October 2000, the *New England Journal of Medicine* (Vol. 343 Issue 17) published a study of AED use by Casino security officers. Of the one hundred-five victims of ventricular fibrillation, fifty-six survived and were discharged from hospital. Ninety patients received the first defibrillation shock in less than five minutes, and on average, the paramedics arrived within ten minutes. They determined a survival rate of almost three in four for those who received their first defibrillation no later than three minutes after a witnessed collapse. It sank to fifty percent for those who were defibrillated after more than three minutes. This is further proof that early access to defibrillation is vital in saving those "hearts too good to die".

AIRLINES

There are as many as one thousand deaths each year due to cardiac arrest on international commercial airline flights. The Federal Aviation Administration ruled that all airliners with at least one flight attendant carry an automated external defibrillator (AED) as standard emergency medical equipment. And, on April 12, 2004, the FAA required AEDs be carried on *all* commercial passenger aircraft of a particular size.

Qantas Airlines was the first airline to install AEDs, starting with their transoceanic flights in 1991. Passenger Roland Koenig made history as the first sudden cardiac arrest victim saved in flight.

American Airlines initiated a program to equip its planes with

AEDs in 1996, and two years later, Robert Giggey of Mebane, North Carolina, became the first AA passenger to be saved, although the plane was still at the gate of Dallas Fort Worth airport. Mike Tighe of Boston Department of Health became the first person saved on a U.S. domestic flight, and is a proud member of the American Airlines Golden Heart Club. In the first two years of the American Airline AED program, over forty percent of the SCA victims (six of fourteen) were resuscitated. This compares with an average SCA survival rate in the United States of just seven percent. By 2003, American Airlines had achieved a fifty-six percent survival rate of the eighty-nine AED events in which a shock was delivered.

In 1999, Singapore Airlines installed defibrillators on all of its eighty-six passenger aircraft, and trained senior cabin crews.

Airliners have a reputation for some of the highest survival rates for cardiac arrest because they are equipped with AEDs and CPR-trained staff, who typically use the devices in a cardiac emergency. It is not too much to hope that other forms of public transport will be just as safe.

AEDs

Almost anyone can learn to operate an AED with a few hours of training, and no medical background is needed. In fact, the American Heart Association advises that, "AEDs are sophisticated, computerized devices that are reliable and simple to operate, enabling lay rescuers with minimal training to administer this lifesaving intervention" (a defibrillation shock), and "flight attendants, security personnel, sports marshals, police officers, firefighters, lifeguards, family members, and many other trained laypersons have used AEDs successfully."

Once an AED is turned on, it provides voice prompts to guide the user through the process. One of the first prompts instructs the user to connect the AED to the victim via the adhesive electrodes (pads) placed on the chest. It then analyzes the victim's heart rhythm through the electrodes, using a built-in computer program, to determine if a shock is required.

If a shock is needed, the AED may prompt the user to press a button that delivers the shock. It will then re-analyze the heart rhythm to determine if more shocks are needed. If a shockable rhythm is not detected, the AED will prompt the user to check the victim for a pulse, and to perform CPR if needed.

AEDs in BUSINESS

Sales of defibrillators to corporations rose thirty-five percent in 2001, as private companies bought over twenty thousand of the automated devices. Some suppliers also provide lease programs, including training, starting at around one hundred dollars per month.

AEDs at HOME

Dr. Bram Zuckerman, director of the FDA's division of cardiovascular devices, indicated that AEDs would be approved for sale without a prescription, after an advisory panel meeting in August 2004. The panel's consensus was that the device, "when used by the intended lay user, is a safe device", and that its effectiveness had been demonstrated. Subsequently, the FDA granted marketing clearance for the first time, for the over-the-counter sale of the HeartStart Home Defibrillator manufactured by Philips Medical Systems. This automatic external defibrillator is designed specifically for lay users, and was already available with a prescription for use at home, but can now be purchased for home use without a prescription.

This century shall see defibrillators, previously operated only by doctors and trained medical staff, become widespread in public buildings, shopping malls, health clubs and schools. In addition, these heart-shockers are now available in the retail market, permitting thousands of untrained Americans to become potential emergency cardiac arrest rescuers.

HEARTY FACTS

If knowledge can create problems,
it is not through ignorance that we can solve them.

—Isaac Asimov

Normal hearts weigh between seven and fifteen ounces, and are a little larger than a fist. If you live past your seventieth birthday your heart will beat more than two billion times without ever pausing to rest. It is a strong, muscular pump that expands and contracts around one hundred thousand times every day, pumping the equivalent of two thousand gallons of blood around your body. It provides the vital ingredients for life itself, and most of the time you will not even notice that it is there.

Your heart has two mechanisms to keep you going; an electrical system and a plumbing system. The plumbing system carries the blood between your lungs and the rest of your body, while the electrical system triggers the heartbeat. And both of them must operate normally to keep you alive. A *cardiac arrest* is usually an electrical problem, while a *heart attack* is usually a plumbing problem. A heart attack, or technically speaking a myocardial infarction (MI), is an example of a plumbing problem caused by clogged or blocked blood vessels that cut off the supply of blood to the heart muscle. The attack typically occurs when that muscle is damaged or destroyed due to a lack of oxygen-rich blood. Just as with the other organs in the body, arterial blood vessels supply oxygen and nutrients to the heart. The heart muscle will be deprived of oxygen if these coronary arteries become blocked or narrowed and, if that oxygen supply is cut off for more than several minutes, the heart cells will suffer permanent damage, or even die.

Myocardial infarctions most often result from coronary heart disease (also called coronary artery disease or ischemic heart disease). The most common cause is atherosclerosis, which is a build-up of fatty deposits called plaque, and commonly known as "hardening of the arteries", since the plaque makes the arterial wall stiff and inflexible. Over time, the plaque clogs and narrows the arteries, which slows or blocks the flow of blood to the heart. Sometimes, the plaque surface will rupture or tear, causing blood clots to form that then block the arteries, a major cause of stroke. A complete or near-complete blockage of the coronary arteries results in a heart attack. Usually, there are warning signs, such as shortness of breath or pain in the chest (often described as crushing or constricting), and possibly cold perspiration.

Heart failure, also called "congestive heart failure", is not specific to either the electrical or plumbing systems. It describes a heart that has become weak and cannot function properly. The name, "heart failure" is confusing, because the heart has not stopped. Instead, one or more chambers of the heart are "failing" to keep up with the demands of the tissues and organs for oxygen-rich blood. Heart enlargement is common in patients with heart failure as the heart muscle expands in an attempt to pump more blood. There is no specific disease; rather, it is a condition or syndrome that is brought on by a variety of underlying diseases or other health problems.

There are two mechanisms that very precisely control your heart rate; the nervous system for instantaneous or short-lived bursts, and hormones, such as epinephrine and norepinephrine, which circulate in the bloodstream and can increase the heart rate for several minutes or more. In people with heart failure, the level of norepinephrine in the blood is chronically elevated in an effort to increase cardiac output by increasing the heart rate.

The nervous system controlling the heart rate has two opposing forces; the sympathetic and parasympathetic. These systems are made up of tiny nerves that connect the brain and spinal cord to your heart. The sympathetic nervous system is triggered during stress or the sudden need for increased cardiac output, and rapidly sends signals to your heart to increase its rate. The parasympathetic system is active during periods of rest, and sends signals to decrease the heart rate, such as during sleep.

༈

The "plumber's" view of the heart is easiest and most commonly understood. The heart is a large and strong, hollow muscle, with four sections called chambers. The heart pumps blood through a sequence of highly organized contractions of the four chambers, with valves to control the flow of blood in and out. Blood flows only one-way around the body, although it is a sixty thousand mile, single-lane highway!

A healthy heart, with normal cardiac output, pumps over a gallon of blood every minute, pushing about a third of a cup of blood in each beat. It starts the journey in the top chambers, called the *atria*, which are the receiving chambers of your heart. When blood flows into your heart from the body or lungs, it always flows into either the right or left atrium (a single upper chamber is called an *atrium*, but when referring to both they are called the atria), which then pushes the blood into the lower chambers. The two lower chambers are the pumping chambers, and are called *ventricles*. When blood leaves your heart, it is always pumped out from the ventricles—strong muscles that create the pressure required to push blood throughout the body.

The right atrium and right ventricle are on the right side of your heart (the same side as your right arm), and the left atrium and left ventricle are on the left side of your heart. When you look at a picture of the heart, however, they are reversed and so right side of the heart is on the left of the picture!

The *septum* is the wall that separates the left and right sides of your heart. Blood that hasn't yet been to the lungs (blood with no oxygen is "blue") stays on the right side of the septum. Blood returning from the lungs (blood with oxygen is "red") stays on the left side of the septum. This seems a little confusing, but is easily remembered by the following; "blue" blood flows from your right atrium into your right ventricle, and "red" blood flows from your left atrium into your left ventricle

Blood flows through each chamber one time on its way through your body—first through the right side of your heart and then through the left. It travels from the upper to the lower chambers, where it is pumped back out to your lungs and body. Your right ventricle pumps the "blue" blood out of your heart to your lungs, where the blood's oxygen supply is replenished. At the same time, the left ventricle pumps "red" blood—once again full of oxygen—out of your heart thru the *aorta* to your body. The aorta is the largest of four major arteries that distributes blood through the body. The pulmonary artery supplies blood to the lungs, and the two coronary arteries bring oxygen rich blood to the heart itself.

❧

An electrician would take a different view of the heart. When working properly, your heart's electrical system automatically responds to your body's changing need for oxygen, by speeding up your heart rate as you climb stairs, for example, or slowing it down when you sleep. When your heart rate increases, it means your heart pumps faster providing more oxygen-rich blood to compensate for the increased demand from your body. This electrical system is quite complex and almost invisible, just as it is in your home. Consider that there are approximately nineteen billion cells in the heart, and to effectively pump blood they must contract in a coordinated fashion. It is almost a miracle, and yet they do it so effortlessly!

There are three major components to the heart's electrical system; the *S-A node*, the *A-V node* and the *His-Purkinje system*. The S-A node (SinoAtrial or sinus node) is the "natural pacemaker" of your heart because it controls your heart rate. It is a bundle of specialized cells in the right atrium that creates the electricity to make your heartbeat. It normally produces sixty to one hundred electrical signals per minute—this is your heart rate, or pulse.

The A-V node (AtrioVentricular) is another bundle of specialized cells between your heart's upper and lower chambers (between the atria and ventricles) that allows the electricity to travel through to the ventricles. This "electrical bridge" passes the electrical trigger from the S-A node to make the ventricles contract and pump the blood around the body. Slow heart rhythms (called *bradycardia*) are sometimes caused by problems in the A-V node.

To give the blood time to flow from the atria into the ventricles the electrical signal from the A-V node is delayed by a fraction of a second. This signal begins its path through the ventricles at the His bundle which then splits into the right bundle branch, and left bundle branch inside the septum, finally ending with the Purkinje fibers (named after the Bohemian physiologist, Jan Evangelista Purkinje, who discovered them in 1839). It takes a certain amount of time, called the QT interval, for the heart's electrical system to recharge after each beat (a process called repolarization), before generating the next signal to activate the contraction of the ventricles. This pattern is most easily recognized in an EKG trace. The first small bump in the rhythm is the P-wave that causes the atria to contract, followed by the big spike of the QRS complex, when the ventricles are energized, and is completed with the round bump that is the repolarizing T-wave.

Problems with these electrical rhythms are numerous, so much so, that they require a cardiac specialist to fully diagnose them. ICDs are programmed to detect and correct the most dangerous of them—the chaotic and extremely rapid beats known as ventricular fibrillation and ventricular tachycardia (generally shortened to V-fib and V-tach).

Typically, electrical rhythm disturbances have an immediate and debilitating effect on the patient, whereas plumbing issues can be slow and gradual—although just as deadly. Any irregular activity in your heart warrants investigation by your doctor, as it is not an organ that tolerates neglect. It has a big job to do and needs the best of care to keep performing.

SHOCKING NUMBERS

The doctor of the future will give no medicine
but will interest his patients in the care of the human frame,
in diet and in the cause and prevention of disease.

–Thomas Edison

Despite the sophisticated engineering of a human heart, more than 1,000 people suddenly die from cardiac arrest each day in the United States alone, *before* they reach a hospital. And over half of them typically had no previous symptoms—nothing to indicate they were in any danger.

The majority of sudden cardiac deaths are caused by ventricular fibrillation, that rapid uncoordinated quivering of the heart's lower chambers, when little or no blood is pumped from the heart. We know there is only an 8-10 minute window of opportunity for a successful rescue—and the greatest chance for survival occurs within the first three minutes. For each minute that passes without defibrillation, survival decreases between seven and ten percent.

Most out-of-hospital sudden cardiac deaths happen at home, but nearly a quarter of them occur in public places where bystanders might be able to help until the emergency medical services arrive.

The Center for Disease Control (CDC) reports that Sudden Cardiac Death (SCD), the *nation's number one killer*, prematurely ended the lives of 460,000 Americans in 1999. Compare that to the number of "more popular deaths": all types of Cancer 550,000, Accidents 101,000, Alzheimer's 53,000, and HIV/AIDS 14,000. More deaths are attributable to SCD than to lung cancer, breast cancer, and AIDS combined.

Now, consider the publicity surrounding road trauma compared to that for SCD. In the United States approximately 40,000 deaths occur annually as a result of motor vehicle accidents, (that is just over 100 per day). Some of them may have been due to SCD, which was possibly the case with Carolyn's father, although he was alone in the car on his way to golf when he died suddenly and no autopsy was performed.

According to the American Heart Association, almost eight million Americans have already survived one heart attack. And there are over 800,000 new heart attack survivors each year. Many of these survivors are at risk for sudden cardiac arrest. In Massachusetts over 15,000 people died from sudden cardiac arrest in 1999, and California takes the record with over 72,000 for the same year. Maybe Rhode Island is a safer community, as only 3,000 died there, and the vast majority were over sixty-five years old.

Another shocking statistic needs to be considered; there were 2,443,930 deaths in the U.S. during 2003, according to the Centers for Disease Control and Prevention. But the overall death rate fell 1.7% from 2002, when adjusted to account for changes in the age distribution of the population. Death rates for the three biggest killers; heart disease, cancer and stroke, also fell between 2.2% and 4.6%. And the average life expectancy in the United States rose to a record 77.6 years in 2003 from 77.3 years in 2002. Women on average live longer than men—80.1 years versus 74.8 years—but the gender gap in mortality has narrowed, continuing a 25-year trend. Are we winning the battle? Could the rescue of more "hearts too good to die" alter these statistics significantly? Surely the prevention of sudden cardiac death by the deployment of AEDs and continuation of CPR training is as important as the research and advanced medical procedures generally attributed to our increased longevity.

Surprisingly, fitness and extraordinary physical capability provides no safety margin. Among athletes, more than 2 in 100,000 people experience sudden death every year, while non-athletes showed a sudden death risk of less than half that rate.

V-fib is just as prevalent worldwide, with a reported predominance in the Northern Hemisphere. Among some European populations, annual incidence of cardiac arrests exceeds 6 per 10,000 people. It has been described as the initial rhythm in almost seventy percent of out-of-hospital arrests, and is the killer in nineteen percent of deaths in pre-teen children, but rises to thirty percent for those aged 14-21 years. (Luckily, there are only around 600 of these cases per year.)

Of the 250,000 patients each year who are newly diagnosed with heart rhythm abnormalities, not all were eligible to receive the devices recommended in American College of Cardiology guidelines. In 2005, the Centers for Medicare and Medicaid Services (CMS) decided to expand coverage to patients warranting ICD therapy, covering as many as 25,000 additional beneficiaries per year. In 1998, there were 26,000 ICD procedures, growing to 46,000 by 2001 in America, (compared to 1.3 million cardiac catheterizations). Each year, more than 175,000 people around the world have a defibrillator implanted in their chest.

❧

Sudden cardiac arrest is a silent killer that, while not often gruesome, is terrifying in its unpredictability. Even Olympic athletes and teenagers have been struck down. Some notable victims include; Hank Gathers, a twenty-three-year-old Loyola Marymount University basketball star who collapsed and died in 1990 during a nationally televised championship game in Los Angeles. There was another basketball star, Reggie Lewis, the twenty-eight-year-old member of the Boston Celtics, who died in 1993 while shooting baskets. Darryl Kile was a thirty-three-year-old baseball pitcher for the St. Louis Cardinals when he collapsed and died in a Chicago hotel room in 2002. In the United Kingdom, Tony Penny, a twenty-three-year-old Central Connecticut State basketball player, collapsed and died in Manchester while playing a professional game in 1990. Anthony Bates was a twenty-year-old Kansas State football player who died of sudden cardiac arrest while driving his car. The Olympic figure skater Sergei Grinkov died during routine practice in 1995, at the age of twenty-eight. Tim Brauch was a twenty-five-year-old professional World Cup skateboarder, ranked fifth internationally, when he suddenly died in 1999. A marathon runner Anna Loyley was twenty-six years old when she died in 1998 after completing the Bath marathon in the United Kingdom. Adam Lemel was a Wisconsin student who collapsed in 1999 during a school basketball game in Milwaukee. Project ADAM (Automatic Defibrillators in Adam's Memory), was created in recognition of the seventeen-year-old, to provide automated external defibrillators in public places, particularly in schools. Mark Barranco, another seventeen-year-old victim, collapsed and died one month later. This Wilmot High School student was also playing basketball. In the same year, a Milwaukee Technical High School football player died of sudden cardiac arrest while playing basketball with friends. Two more Milwaukee-area deaths were recorded in 2000; a Marquette University senior, and a visiting 12-year-old baseball player from Illinois.

Not all the stories are distressing, however. Just as Carolyn was saved, there are many more survivors, and hopefully we can reverse the ratio of lost to living. Kayla Burt was a twenty-one-year-old sophomore who suffered a cardiac arrest on New Year's Eve, 2002, and now has a defibrillator implanted in her chest. Paul Arcangeli was thirty-three in 1999 when he collapsed at 3am. The United States Army bomb disposal officer was an avid runner in good shape, and faced the dangers of his job with courage. Now he has an ICD to remind him of his mortality. Kindel VanCronkhite died in 1999, but her twenty-four-year-old twin sister soon had an ICD implanted to protect her. Tragically they had had a first cousin die of sudden cardiac death in 1994. And there is, of course, Vice President Dick Cheney, who, after surviving a heart attack in 2001, received an ICD because his cardiologists determined his risk of sudden cardiac death was high.

෴

Fortunately, the statistics are not all bad. Survivors of a sudden cardiac arrest have an excellent prognosis: 83% survive for at least one year, and 57% survive for five years or longer. In fact, when analyzed by age group, survival rates for sudden cardiac arrest survivors are comparable to survival rates of people who have never had an event.

Undeniably, early intervention and application of the "chain of survival" including defibrillation and ICD implantation can offer years of productivity and fulfillment to victims of sudden cardiac arrest.

CHAPTER NOTES

When you know a thing, to hold that you know it;
and when you do not know a thing,
to allow that you do not know it;
this is knowledge.

–Confucius

In many places I have avoided explaining in detail the reasoning and background to the medical procedures or emergency care protocols described. These notes fill in those details that might otherwise distract you from the story. When reading I often find myself asking questions of the author as I enter their written world. I hope you do too, and that you will use the following pages for some of the answers.

CHAPTER ONE

What Does "Critical Condition" Mean?

In Carolyn's case it meant, "uncertain prognosis, vital signs are abnormal, and death may be imminent."

Under HIPAA, hospital personnel are advised to use one-word answers to describe patient conditions, as documented in the *General Guide for the Release of Information on the Condition of Patients*:

Undetermined:	Patient awaiting physician and assessment.
Critical:	Vital signs are unstable and not within normal limits. Patient may not be conscious. Indicators are unfavorable.
Serious:	Vital signs unstable or not within normal limits. Patient is acutely ill. Indicators are questionable.
Fair:	Vital signs are stable and within normal limits. Patient is conscious, possibly uncomfortable. Indicators are favorable.
Good:	Vital signs are stable and within normal limits. Patient is conscious and comfortable. Indicators are excellent.

The term "vital signs" describes indicators such as blood pressure, pulse, temperature, and respiration.

What is CPR and how does it help?

Cardiopulmonary resuscitation (CPR) is a life saving first aid procedure for assisting unconscious patients before emergency medical help arrives, and is essential if there is no pulse.

Depriving a person's brain of oxygen for only a few seconds will cause unconsciousness, and starts an irreversible sequence of destruction. Restoring the oxygen supply to the brain is crucial to a successful resuscitation. Oxygen can only be transferred to the brain cells via the bloodstream, so restoring circulation is vital. Without a pulse or breathing, a person will die within four or five minutes.

CPR follows the simple algorithm of ABC: Airway, Breathing, and Circulation. Almost anyone can perform the tasks, and it is often taught in schools and first aid courses. CPR ensures that there is air for the lungs and that blood flows to the brain and lungs, by forcing air into the mouth, and compressing the heart (pushing down on the chest) to pump the blood. It is best performed with two people, one for the air and the other for the compressions. At the very least, compressions are essential, since they also tend to move air in and out of the lungs.

Both the AHA and the Red Cross have highly successful education programs for teaching CPR.

What did those EMT guys do to Carolyn?

The average response time to an emergency call is six to twelve minutes. In cities like New York, there can be a significant delay between a 9-1-1 call and the response, especially if the EMTs have to enter a multi-story building. In Carolyn's case, the hotel security staff were trained and prepared to direct the EMTs directly to the conference room.

ENDOTRACHEAL INTUBATION is used to secure an open airway in patients that cannot maintain their own airway. A plastic tube is inserted through the mouth and into the lungs, then a ventilation bag is attached and pumped by hand, or the tube is connected to an oxygen bottle with a regulator that will deliver a constant pressure into the lungs. Intubation also helps prevent aspiration, where contents of the stomach or throat can be forced into the lungs, causing blockages and infection.

The LIFEPAK®12 Defibrillator/Monitor is manufactured by Medtronic and is designed specifically for EMS and hospital use. It weighs less than five pounds and provides paramedics with access to sophisticated diagnostics and treatment in the field. With a five-inch LCD display and Continuous Patient Surveillance System (CPSS), this single piece of equipment monitors the ECG continuously, measures the level of oxygen in the bloodstream and, if necessary, provides defibrillation and pacing to help maintain the heart's rhythm. The unit has a typical charge time to 360 Joules of less than ten seconds and is powered by Ni-Cad batteries or AC mains electricity.

In the field, they typically use disposable electrode pads (Medtronic brand name Fast-Patch) that both measure the heart activity and deliver the electrical stimulation to shock the heart back into normal rhythm. There are usually several shocks administered. The first one "polarizes" the heart to reduce the chest impedance (resistance to electricity), and subsequent ones remove the life threatening fibrillation, but each time at a higher energy level. Most AEDs deliver three consecutive jolts preset to 200J, 200J, and 360J.

Why is defibrillation necessary?
Ventricular fibrillation eventually deteriorates into a total absence of electrical activity around ten to fifteen minutes after arrest. This is because once the blood flow to the heart muscle stops, the cells begin to lose the energy to contract, and will not recover even if blood flow is restored.

The best chance to regain a pulse is when a patient in VF is shocked quickly—ideally within 4-6 minutes after arrest. When an AED delivers a shock, it causes an electrical current to pass through the heart muscle, temporarily ceasing all electrical activity in the heart. The intention is that when the natural electrical impulse returns, the heart will return to an organized pumping action instead of VF.

When the heart stops pumping blood, one of the organs most affected is the heart itself. The hypoxia, lack of oxygen, interferes with the electrical functions of the ventricles. This can affect the ability of the heart to resume normal sinus rhythm once the defibrillator has overpowered the chaotic rhythm. Thus, the heart muscle often needs powerful drugs to encourage normal myocardial cell functions.

EPINEPHRINE is used for improving the blood flow to the heart and brain by up to fifteen times during CPR. It is the drug of first choice for patients without a pulse, and makes the CPR more effective. This hormone, also known as adrenaline, is naturally produced in the adrenal gland. The name comes from the Greek "upon kidney"; *epi* + *nephros*.

1:10000 IV push means intravenous injection of one milligram of the drug diluted to one in ten thousand with a saline solution.

CORDARONE (also called Amiodarone) is a "broad spectrum" antiarrhythmic medication. It has multiple and complex effects on the heart's electrical activity and is used to correct irregular heartbeats. It operates by slowing down the nerve impulses in the heart, delaying the recharge after contraction (repolarization). This prolongs the stimulation of the heart muscle cells, and reduces the heart's natural pacemaker firing rate. In addition, it causes the blood vessels to dilate (enlarge) which can also result in a drop in blood pressure.

LIDOCAINE is an anti-fibrillation drug to help the heart muscle regain a normal electrical rhythm. Its anti-arrhythmic properties increase the electrical stimulation threshold of the ventricles, suppressing the automaticity of conduction through the tissue, and thereby reduce premature ventricular contractions. It is also widely used as a local anesthetic.

The term BOLUS refers to a single dose of drug usually injected into a blood vessel over a short period of time.

Which hospital is the best one?
If you're seriously hurt or ill, you want to go to a hospital that is very busy. The ER staffs are quick to respond and very experienced, as opposed to an emergency room that has never dealt with the problem before. Obviously, the closest ER is the best in a life or death situation.
What were those blood tests?
CBC: Complete Blood Count reveals the oxygen carrying capacity of the blood, and can indicate foreign cell invasion (i.e. bacteria) or drugs. This test is commonly used with cardiac patients to provide a baseline for evaluation of treatment, and to test for evidence of internal bleeding.

CMP: Comprehensive Metabolic Panel gives insight into the condition of kidneys, liver, electrolytes and acid/base balance, blood sugar and blood proteins

CPK, CK-MB: Creatine Kinase (CK) is one of the cellular enzymes released into the blood after irreversible cell injury. It can indicate cardiac (MB), cerebral (BB) or skeletal (MM) muscle damage, and is often used to confirm the clinical diagnosis of myocardial infarction.

ABG; Arterial Blood Gas is used to measure the oxygen and carbon dioxide levels in the blood leaving the heart.

CHAPTER TWO
What are smalls?
This is an old-fashioned, informal plural noun of UK origins that describes underwear, especially when being washed or about to be washed: Have you got any smalls that need washing?
ANEURISM (aneurysm): A bulging out of part of the wall of a blood vessel. It forms where the wall has weakened, often due to the build-up of plaque. It may also be an inherited condition, or a complication of high blood pressure (hypertension). If left untreated, aneurisms may tear or burst (a ruptured aneurism). Some aneurisms rupture without any warning signs at all, and are very painful events that cause massive internal bleeding. Cerebral aneurism can cause stroke and paralysis. Survivors of a ruptured aneurism are initially at increased risk of

developing abnormal heart rhythms. Fortunately, Carolyn did not have an aneurism or a stroke, unlike Robert McCrum, who describes the terrifying consequences in his book, *My Year Off.*

CHAPTER THREE

Special equipment is used to help recovery in the ICU, including the following:

- Ventilator or respirator; an artificial breathing machine provides oxygen at a constant volume and constant pressure, and pushes air in and out of the lungs through an endotracheal tube. The mix of air and oxygen, as well as the volume and pressure can be adjusted. The endotracheal tube in the windpipe can increase the risk of bacterial infections and the pressures used with a ventilator can be damaging to the lung tissues.

- Intravenous (IV) catheter; a plastic tube with needle that is inserted through the skin into blood vessels to provide IV fluids and medications.

- Nasogastric (NG) tube; a small, clear, flexible tube that keeps the stomach drained of acid and gas bubbles that may build up in unconscious patients.

- Urinary catheter; a thin, flexible tube that permits urine to drain out of the bladder to be captured. Accurately measuring how much urine the body produces helps determine cardiac health. When the heart function is abnormal, the body often retains fluids, causing swelling and puffiness. Diuretics may be given to help the kidneys remove these excess fluids from the body.

- Heart monitor; a machine connected via patches on the chest and back to measure the tiny electrical signals within the heart. It constantly displays a picture of the heart rhythm. Usually this one device monitors heart rate, arterial blood pressure, blood oxygen level and other critical values.

HEART ATTACK: More properly known as a myocardial infarction (MI), because part of the heart muscle (myocardium) may literally die (infarction), and generally occurs when part of the heart is not getting enough oxygen-rich blood (cardiac ischemia). Small attacks maybe undetected, but over time the cumulative effects of this damage can lead to heart failure.

ECHOCARDIOGRAM: A painless, non-invasive, safe and very accurate test to study the anatomy of the heart. It uses sound waves (ultrasound or "echo") to create a moving picture of your heart, similar to the ultrasounds used for pregnancies. The patient lies down, while a transducer (a device like a computer mouse) is moved back and forth across the chest, collecting several "views" to form images of the structures of the heart. The test takes between thirty to sixty minutes, and determines the size, shape, thickness and movement of the chambers of the heart, the quality of the valves, and ultimately measures the heart's pumping ability. It can also determine if there is fluid, blood clots or tumors in specific areas of the heart.

Why was she paralyzed?

MIDAZOLAM: Used for patients in intensive care units to cause unconsciousness. This can help reduce the stress of mechanically assisted breathing, and aids the recovery from trauma.

CHAPTER FOUR

BLOOD OXYGEN LEVELS: When the amount of oxygen supplied by the blood declines, the brain cells cannot keep up with the demand for energy. At a critically low level of oxygen, the energy in neurons becomes so low that there is no interneuronal (between neurons) electrical communication and the patient may lose consciousness. At a low enough level, the cells cannot maintain their internal fluid balance, causing swelling, failure of metabolism, and ultimately, cell death. If enough neurons in a functionally significant area of the brain die, the patient will have a permanent neurological disability (i.e., a stroke).

Arterial oxygen levels are usually 95% or more. Below a level of 80%, the cells do not receive enough oxygen to continue to function normally. At 30% saturation, the cells are dying. The degree of damage from low oxygen saturation depends on how long the cells are "de-saturated". Unfortunately, some of the more serious cell damage due to low oxygen (hypoxia) or no oxygen (anoxia) is irreversible. Even neurons that are not quite dead after an episode of a few minutes' anoxia will die even if normal oxygen supply (and saturation) is restored.

INTRAVENOUS FLUIDS: Given in large quantities to heart damage victims to increase the blood volume, and thus help to maintain a good blood pressure.

Unfortunately, a nasty side effect of these IV fluids is the swelling and puffiness they cause in the body tissues. Additionally, when the cardiac function is abnormal, the body often retains fluids through the release of aldosterone, which also causes swelling and puffiness. Plasma electrolyte imbalances can have a profound effect on cardiovascular function, especially myocardial contraction. One condition called hypokalemia—a decrease in potassium concentration—can contribute to arrhythmia through hyperpolarization of the myocardial cells.

HEPARIN: A natural product (originally isolated from liver cells, but now made synthetically). This colorless to slightly yellow solution is used as an anticoagulant (slowing the rate of blood clot formation), and is sometimes called a blood thinner, although it does not actually thin the blood. Technically, it is used as a prophylactic measure (to prevent, rather than treat or cure) against thrombosis (formation of a clot or thrombus inside a blood vessel). Carolyn was administered heparin as a preventative measure, as they suspected there were blocked arteries stopping the blood flow to her heart. This was the ICU doctor's best guess as to the cause of her cardiac arrest, but it was later proven not to be the case.

BLOOD PRESSURE: Most often read using a sphygmomanometer (a gauge attached to a rubber cuff which is wrapped around the upper arm), and a stethoscope. The cuff is inflated to the point where the pulse is no longer heard, and then the pressure is slowly released. The pressure at which the heartbeat is first heard is called the SYSTOLIC pressure, and indicates the maximum arterial pressure during contraction of the left ventricle of the heart. In a blood pressure reading, the systolic pressure is typically the first number recorded. The DIASTOLIC pressure is the minimum arterial pressure during relaxation and dilatation of the ventricles of the heart when the ventricles fill with blood. It is the second number recorded.

Systolic comes from the Greek *systole* meaning "a drawing together or a contraction." Diastolic also comes from the Greek—*diastole* meaning "a drawing apart." The terms have been in use since the 16th century to denote the periods of contraction and relaxation of the heart muscle. The word sphygmomanometer (pronounced sfig·mo·ma·nom·e·ter) was put together from the Greek *sphygmos*, the beating of the heart or the pulse + *manometer*, a device for measuring pressure or tension.

Why do they measure the liquid output?
Reduced urine output is an indicator of cardiogenic shock (dramatic reduction in blood pressure and blood flow), which can lead to V-fib, due to the acidosis from lack of oxygen. When the cells in the body do not get enough oxygen to function, they start an alternative metabolism that produces lactic acid (instead of carbon dioxide which is removed by the lungs), and this builds up in the blood. Acidosis is dangerous because it increases the electrical instability of the heart muscle.

CHAPTER FIVE
ANGIOGRAM: This procedure provides a visual indication of the health of coronary arteries. A contrast material that can be seen using x-ray equipment is injected into one of the arteries via a catheter inserted in the groin. The resulting "photographs" can show blockages or bulges in the arteries. It is a relatively safe procedure, but does involve piercing an artery and feeding a long tube inside the blood vessel and into the heart.

CHAPTER SIX
EP STUDY: This procedure records the speed and flow of the heart's electrical signals from the inside of the ventricles and atria, using

catheters fed along the blood vessels into the heart chambers. The catheters are positioned at various locations in the heart, using the real time x-ray capabilities of a fluoroscope, so that electrical signals can be recorded from each of the locations simultaneously. The catheters can also serve as pacemakers that allow the electrophysiologist to stimulate the heart and initiate an arrhythmia. This helps to pinpoint the areas in the heart that may be the sources of abnormal electrical signals that could trigger ventricular fibrillation. The physician can also determine if a patient has had a heart attack without knowing it, and can detect the evidence of prior heart damage. The study maps the location of the specific section of the heart that produces the arrhythmia. In some cases, the electrophysiologist may attempt to destroy some of the tissue, using radiofrequency ablation techniques, so that the arrhythmia cannot recur.

What are "Advance Directives"?

Advance directives—a living will, or health care power of attorney—allow you to give instructions about your future medical care should you be unable to do so yourself when the need arises. By making your wishes clear, advance directives can help spare your family the burden of trying to guess what medical care you would want in a particular situation. Affected only if you are near death, and unable to communicate, advance directives let you document the forms of medical treatment acceptable to you (within the bounds of state law). A health care power of attorney lets you appoint a trusted individual (sometimes called your proxy or agent) to make health care decisions for you if you are incapacitated, even if you are not terminally ill or near death.

CAPSULAR TISSUE: Capsules of living, tightly woven collagen fibers naturally form around a foreign body, such as titanium ICD implants. The capsule is thought to form in order to shield the body from the foreign object by creating a fibrous wall of tissue, to separate them and prevent friction within the body cavity.

Carolyn's ICD details

The Medtronic Gem III VR defibrillation system is highly effective at accurately detecting ventricular tachyarrhythmias and delivering three different types of therapies to stop ventricular tachyarrhythmia episodes.

1. Fast pacing (anti-tachycardia pacing) to overdrive the tachyarrhythmia and allow the heart to resume a more normal rate. Most ventricular tachycardia episodes are stopped by this first-line of therapy. Patients report that this therapy is not felt.

2. Cardioversion therapy that delivers a measured shock at a specific point in the heartbeat cycle to reset the tachyarrhythmia to a more normal rate. Many episodes that are not stopped by fast pacing can be stopped by cardioversion. This shock will be felt.

3. Defibrillation that delivers an immediate full-strength shock to reset the tachyarrhythmia. Nearly all episodes can be stopped by defibrillation. This shock is definitely felt, like a kick in the chest, but it is necessary to stop the episode.

The five stages of grief

Elisabeth Kubler-Ross, in her book *On Death and Dying*, outlined the stages that terminally ill patients go through in coping with the devastating knowledge of their ailment. The now popular term "five stages of grief" is attributed to this book, but Kubler-Ross's description is better: "The five stages of receiving catastrophic news". I have witnessed friends and family going through this process when a sudden and unexpected change occurred, such as a separation, divorce, death or other form of loss. The five stages Kubler-Ross defined are: Denial, Anger, Bargaining, Depression, and Acceptance. In my opinion, emotions are so complex that not all stages become evident, and will not necessarily follow in that order.

CHAPTER NINE

There are two major classes of Ambulance service:

Basic Life Support (BLS). A person trained to provide BLS services is usually certified as an Emergency Medical Technician (EMT). Most ambulance service personnel are trained to this level, and form the backbone of the emergency medical system. EMTs provide a level of care including patient assessment, CPR, bandaging, splinting broken bones, administration of oxygen, and defibrillation.

Advanced Life Support (ALS). Generally, paramedic programs provide ALS training that includes defibrillation, administering IV medications, cardiac monitoring, and advanced airway management. Paramedics are certified to provide care to emergency patients in out-of-hospital settings.

First responders are generally not equipped or trained in the use of AEDs, but this situation is being addressed, as the awareness of SCD increases, and the cost of defibrillators declines.

BRAIN DAMAGE is most often due to a lack of oxygen, from either hypoxia or anoxia. The brain cells store a very small amount of oxygen, which is typically exhausted in less than twenty seconds. This causes disruption to the delicate chemical balance between the inside and outside of the cells. Calcium starts to build up inside the cell, and a chemical chain reaction begins to destroy the genetic material inside the nucleus, causing irreversible damage to the cell. As the genetic code that regulates all the activity in a cell breaks down, it releases acids into the bloodstream, causing even more damage. This acid level will plateau within fifteen minutes.

Sugar is just as important as oxygen, and is also stored in the cells. After five minutes of no blood flow, this glucose is depleted, depriving the brain cells of the energy to fuel the chemical reactions, accelerating the cell destruction. The critical period for restoration of oxygen to the brain is before these destructive processes occur—five minutes for the sugars and fifteen minutes for the acid levels. Once the process begins inside the cells, they will not recover, and irreversible brain damage will have occurred.

CHAPTER TEN

Permission received for reprinting material from *Thriving with Heart Disease*, Wayne M. Sotile, Ph.D., (Free Press 2003). (p. 225)

SHOCKING NUMBERS

SCA claims more lives each year than these other diseases combined:

40,600 - Breast Cancer - American Cancer Society, 2001

42,156 - AIDS - U.S. Census Bureau, Statistical Abstract of the U. S., 2001

157,400 - Lung Cancer -American Cancer Society, 2001

167,366 - Stroke - 2002Heart and Stroke Statistical Update, AHA

450,000 - SCA - Circulation. 2001; 104:2158-2163

Other causes of death:

Automobile accident - 50,000 - National Transportation Safety Board, 2000

Fires - 4,000 - NFPA, U.S. Facts & Figures, 2000

Source of statistics: AHA, Heart Disease and Stroke Statistics, 2004 Update

Source of athletic statistics: Journal of the American College of Cardiology, 2003

GLOSSARY OF MEDICAL TERMINOLOGY AND PROCEDURES

Internists know everything and do nothing,
Surgeons know nothing and do everything,
Dermatologists know nothing and do nothing,
Pathologists know everything and do everything—but always too late.

ANGIOGRAM

Sometimes called an arteriogram, since it is effectively taking pictures of the arteries. It can be used to examine almost any artery, including those of the head, kidneys, heart, or lungs. For the heart, it is called coronary angiography, and is usually performed to detect obstructions in the coronary arteries that can lead to heart attack. An angiogram involves three major steps: 1) insertion of a catheter (small tube) into your blood vessels, 2) taking x-ray pictures while a contrast (radioactive dye) is injected into the artery, and 3) removal of the catheter. The results are often a "photo" of the inside of your arteries, similar to an x-ray film.

ANOXIA & HYPOXIA

Anoxia (absence of oxygen in arterial blood or the tissues) is a condition in which there is no oxygen supply to an organ's tissues, although there may be adequate blood flow to the tissue.

Hypoxia (depletion of oxygen in the cells) describes the condition in which the blood is carrying abnormally low levels of oxygen.

ARRHYTHMIA

In very simple terms, an arrhythmia is an abnormal heart rhythm resulting from electrical instability within the heart muscle. The abnormal heartbeat may be unusually fast (tachycardia) or unusually slow (bradycardia). It may be related to a previous heart condition (e.g., damage from a heart attack) or to other factors like caffeine, stress or medications.

Any change from the normal sequence of electrical impulses will cause abnormal heart rhythms, or arrhythmia. This can cause the heart to pump less effectively, sometimes so briefly that the overall heart rate and rhythm isn't greatly affected. Examples include; a temporary pause, premature beats, or premature ventricular contractions. Arrhythmias that continue for too long may cause the heart rhythm to become erratic.

The most deadly cardiac rhythm disturbance is ventricular fibrillation (VF or V-fib), a condition when the lower chambers (the ventricles) quiver and the heart can't pump any blood at all, resulting in death within a few minutes. (Ventricular Asystole is even more dangerous as it is caused by complete failure of the electrical connection to the ventricles and may not respond to defibrillation. This condition is fairly rare, but is often displayed in TV shows as a flat line and continuous beep/tone. It is also a sign of death.)

CARDIOMYOPATHY

Cardiomyopathy is a type of progressive disease of the heart muscle in which the heart is abnormally enlarged, thickened and/or stiffened. People with this genetic heart disease are at increased risk for sudden cardiac death, since the heart cannot pump blood as well as it should.

CARDIOVERSION

Cardioversion can be chemical or electrical. Chemical cardioversion refers to the use of anti-arrhythmia medications to restore the heart's normal rhythm. Anti-arrhythmia medications work by modifying the heart's electrical properties to reduce the frequency of abnormal heart rhythms, and to help restore a normal rhythm. One drug that is often used is called amiodarone (brand name Cordorone). Electrical cardioversion refers to the use of a short, sharp electrical shock to interrupt the abnormal rhythm, allowing the heartbeat to resume by itself. Defibrillation is the strongest form of cardioversion.

CARDIOPULMONARY RESUCITATION (CPR) TRAINING

When a bystander performs CPR, the victim's chance of surviving a sudden cardiac arrest is tripled. More than half the adult population in America has participated in CPR classes.

Firefighters work as instructors for the Seattle program, and teach about 18,000 people a year. Since 1971, the city has trained 650,000 people. As a result, Seattle now has one of the highest bystander CPR rates in the nation—44%. This means that nearly half of all cardiac arrest victims get CPR from a co-worker, a loved one or a stranger in the minutes between collapse and the arrival of an emergency medical team.

Boston's bystander CPR rate is 30%; that is, bystanders are already performing CPR when rescue crews arrive in nearly one out of three cases. The city has saved more than 200 lives over the past decade with a public training program conducted by the fire department.

Two key findings from recent studies in Michigan and Sweden are; 1) In cities where CPR training is widespread and EMS response is rapid, the survival rate increased from 7% to 26% when AEDs were available to first responders; 2) In cities where defibrillation is provided within 5 to 7 minutes, the survival rate from cardiac arrest was as high as 49%.

In summary, CPR keeps a heart quivering. Victims are more often found still in V-fib by medics when a bystander performs CPR. Without CPR they die. In addition, strangers *will* come to the rescue. Victims are four times more likely to get bystander CPR outside the home than inside.

DEFIBRILLATION

You have probably seen a defibrillator used on TV shows like ER and General Hospital. A physician, a paddle in each hand, yells, "Clear!" while applying the paddles to the chest of a patient, and shocks the patient "back to life". During fibrillation, the heart cells are not contracting in synchrony, but fire randomly, causing the heart to quiver ineffectively. Without intervention to get the cells contracting in unison, death is certain.

Defibrillation (or electrical cardioversion) is an electric shock therapy that attempts to depolarize the heart muscle, and thus allows the SA Node to resume its normal pacemaker function. The shock causes all the heart cells to contract simultaneously, thereby interrupting and terminating the abnormal electrical rhythm without damaging the heart.

ECG

An electrocardiogram or ECG (also called an EKG) is a common, painless test that records the rate and regularity of heartbeats, by measuring the tiny electrical signals with electrodes placed on the patient's skin (usually on the chest, but sometimes also the arms and legs). An ECG can tell if the heart is beating normally. It can detect problems with the electrical system of the heart, as well as the effects of drugs or devices such as pacemakers and ICDs.

The ECG machine records the electrical activity of the heart and converts it into lines, called waveforms, which can be seen on a monitor or printed on paper strip. A standard ECG test records the heart rhythm for 12 seconds. All ECG machines operate at the same speed, so the squares on the paper represent time, with the printed waveforms measuring the rate of movement of the heart's electrical impulses. These impulses are shown as a series of waves and complexes called the P wave, the QRS complex, the T wave and the U wave. A normal heartbeat has waves separated by regular intervals. When the intervals are not regular, it may be a sign of heart disease or other problems like arrhythmia.

ECHOCARDIOGRAM

These tests use ultrasound—very high frequency sound waves—to inspect the structure and function of the heart. A transducer (a microphone-like device) sends a beam of sound waves through the patient's chest wall to the heart. When the beam hits the different types of tissue in the heart it is reflected back through to the transducer according to the various densities of those tissues. The amount of time the waves take to travel through the tissue and back to the transducer is analyzed and determines the size, shape, thickness and movement of the different structures in the heart. A moving image of the patient's beating heart is displayed on a video monitor, where the cardiologist can study the heart's thickness, size and function. The image also shows the motion-pattern and structure of the four heart valves, revealing any potential leakage (regurgitation). A Doppler ultrasound may also be undertaken to evaluate blood flow through the heart valves.

EJECTION FRACTION (EF)

This measure of heart function determines the proportion, or fraction, of blood pumped out of your heart with each beat, and is measured during an echocardiogram. A normal heart will pump out about 55% of the blood in the ventricles. A damaged heart that is at risk for cardiac arrest typically has an EF of 35% or lower.

ELECTROPHYSIOLOGIST

Cardiologists who have additional education and training in the diagnosis and treatment of abnormal heart rhythms are called electrophysiologists. Electrophysiology is the fastest growing of all the cardiovascular disciplines.

EP STUDY

An electrophysiology study is key to diagnosing and treating arrhythmias and can help predict if an individual is at high risk for sudden cardiac death. The electrophysiologist provokes arrhythmia events to locate the specific areas of heart tissue that give rise to abnormal electrical impulses.

During the study, the physician studies the speed and flow of electrical signals through the heart, identifies rhythm problems, and pinpoints areas in the heart that give rise to abnormal electrical signals. To measure the electrical impulses, a catheter with monitoring electrodes is inserted through a vein or artery into the heart, from a site in the groin or neck. The journey from entry point to heart muscle is navigated by images created by a fluoroscope, an x-ray-like machine that provides "live" images of the catheter and heart muscle.

This test is performed in a safe and controlled electrophysiology laboratory at a hospital or clinic. The patient is in little danger and complications are rare. The procedure takes about two hours; the patient is given local anesthesia and conscious sedation (twilight sleep), but is awake and must remain still.

HEART RHYTHMS

Bradycardia describes a heartbeat that is too slow (less than sixty beats a minute). The weak pace may mean the heart doesn't beat often enough to ensure adequate blood flow. Slow heart rates can be the result of certain medications, congenital heart disease, or the degenerative processes of aging. Heart block (or AV Block) and Sick Sinus Syndrome are forms of bradycardia.

Tachycardia (tachy means fast) is a too-rapid heartbeat. There are two predominant types of tachycardia: supraventricular tachycardia (SVT) and ventricular tachycardia (VT). The most common type of SVT is atrial fibrillation, an irregular and rapid heartbeat in the upper chambers of the heart (or atria). More than two million people in the United States have atrial fibrillation, and 160,000 new cases are diagnosed each year. It is not a deadly arrhythmia, but can cause a stroke by the formation of clots in the atria. At times, ventricular tachycardia (VT) can change without warning into the deadly arrhythmia, *ventricular fibrillation* (VF). Rapid, irregular and chaotic heartbeats in the lower chambers of the heart (or ventricles) are a sign of ventricular fibrillation. Within seconds, the victim loses consciousness and will die within minutes, without immediate emergency defibrillation.

HOLTER MONITORS, EVENT MONITORS

These are external devices that are worn by an individual who may be at risk for heart disease. The monitor automatically records a continuous electrocardiogram (ECG) of the heart's electrical activity, and is usually worn for 24 to 48 hours. An event recorder is a small, pager-sized device that also records the electrical activity of the heart. Unlike a Holter monitor, it does not operate continuously, but instead is activated by the individual whenever he or she feels the heart begin to beat too fast or chaotically. After the device is activated to record the heart rhythm, the patient can report the event by transmitting the recording via telephone.

HYPERTROPHIC CARDIOMYOPATHY (HCM)

Hypertrophic refers to an abnormal growth of muscle fibers in the heart muscle. Cardiomyopathy is the disease in which the heart is abnormally enlarged, thickened and/or stiffened.

Therefore Hypertrophic Cardiomyopathy (HCM) describes the thickening of the heart muscle, most commonly at the septum, below the aortic valve, and in the left ventricle.

HYPOXIA and ANOXIA

The terms anoxia and hypoxia are often used interchangeably—without regard to their specific meanings—to describe a condition that occurs in an organ when there is a diminished supply of oxygen.

"In severe cases of anoxia and hypoxia, from any cause, the patient is often stuperous or comatose (in a state of unconsciousness) for periods ranging from hours to days, weeks, or months. Seizures, myoclonic jerks (muscle spasms or twitches), and neck stiffness may occur." (*Healthlink*, Medical College of Wisconsin.)

IMPLANTABLE CARDIOVERTER DEFIBRILLATOR (ICD)

A small, fully implantable, battery-operated device, about the size of a stopwatch. Generally placed under the skin just below the collarbone, and connected by special wires (electrode leads) to the heart muscle. The electrode touches the inside of the heart wall (inside the right ventricle) making a secure electrical contact for the pulse generator that delivers the electrical shock.. The system is designed to recognize and terminate ventricular tachyarrhythmias and to deliver a lifesaving jolt of electricity directly to the heart to restore a normal rhythm. It is effective in fighting cardiac arrest over ninety percent of the time.

These sophisticated medical devices have advanced a long way from 1985, when FDA approval was first granted. The first generation ICDs, introduced in the early 1980s, were implanted in the abdomen, as they were so big and bulky. They were also short lived, compared with the fourth generation units now small enough to be implanted under the skin just above the left breast and designed to last for many years. Tens of thousands of Americans have had fourth generation units installed. These tiny digital computers, with on board memory are not much bigger than a pacemaker, but are designed to detect deadly arrhythmias and deliver the life saving shocks with extreme precision and reliability.

The electrode leads are designed to be durable and reliable, and are composed of one continuous piece of silicone tubing with an extendable/retractable screw-in tip that holds the discharge coils in the correct location inside the heart.

A typical shock drains about two weeks of energy from the ICD battery, and many devices have a low-battery warning feature. They will beep or produce a steady tone like an alarm clock when less than six months of battery life remains.

ICDs keep a record of any abnormal heart rhythms, especially dangerous waveforms, for analysis by an electrophysiologist after the event. Some ICDs are also programmed to "pace" the heart to restore a natural rhythm much like a pacemaker.

The cardiac electrical problems that an ICD of dead tissue protects against are usually irreversible, and incurable for the foreseeable future. Thus, an ICD is implanted forever, although in reality they are replaced every decade or so, as the battery wears out and improved models are developed. ICDs are greatly superior to drug therapy for treatment of sustained arrhythmia events, and are essential for patients at risk of sudden cardiac arrest.

Many patients suffering sudden cardiac arrests have had a heart attack in the past. Heart attacks increase the risk of fibrillation because they leave scars inside the heart. This scar tissue has a higher electrical resistance and disturbs the electrical pathway, causing arrhythmias.

INTRAVENOUS (IV) LINES

A catheter that is inserted into a vein (intravenous) is considered when a person requires frequent or continuous injections of medications and fluids.

The typical "hospital IV" line put in your hand or forearm when you are admitted to the hospital is called a Peripheral Venous Access (in the arm). It is a short catheter, usually less than one inch long, that is inserted into a small peripheral vein, and is meant to be temporary. These catheters need to be changed every three days, or more often if they dislodge from the vein. Many medications can irritate peripheral veins because they are thin and have a small amount of blood flowing past the catheter. There is usually a plastic dressing over the catheter to keep it clean and dry at all times. Blood cannot be drawn for lab tests from a peripheral catheter, and it needs to be flushed with a saline and heparin injection after every use or at least twice daily if not in use. Saline is a salt solution used to clean or "flush out" the catheter, and heparin is flushed into the catheter to prevent the blood clotting between uses.

A central line (or central catheter) is usually placed in the subclavian vein—the Superior Vena Cava. Generally made of polymeric silicone rubber, they are extremely flexible and soft, and should be treated gently. A Dacron felt cuff anchors the catheter in place subcutaneously, sealing the junction and preventing bacteria from crawling along the outside of the catheter into the blood stream. Two popular brand names of this type of catheter are Hickman® and Groshong®. The Groshong catheters have a pressure-sensitive, two-way valve at the tip, preventing backflow of blood into the catheter, and so clamping and frequent heparin flushing is not as necessary.

Central Catheters with multiple lumens are commonly used instead of a peripheral catheter because they offer greater versatility than using a Y-connector for connecting numerous lines. Specific lumens can be assigned for drug infusion and the remaining lumen, usually color-coded red, is used for blood aspiration for lab tests.

The advantage of a permanent central venous catheter is that it avoids the need for frequent intravenous catheters in the arm. Many of the medications and nutritional fluids a person requires are too damaging to the smaller veins in the arms to allow for their administration in that manner.

Central venous catheters are almost always done with local anesthetic and intravenous sedation. The procedure is relatively safe, and has few complications. Short-term complications are related to placement of a needle into the vein through which the catheter is threaded. It is possible for the needle to puncture a lung or cause bleeding into the chest. Long-term complications include clotting of blood inside the catheter and catheter infections.

ISCHEMIA

This term simply means deprived of oxygen, and describes a condition where the oxygen-rich blood flow to a part of the body is restricted, often due to obstruction in an artery. The term is usually used in conjunction with an organ or tissue, i.e., ischemic stroke.

MAGNET MODE

This is a feature of ICDs, which is activated when a magnet is placed over the pulse generator of the ICD. In general, magnet mode is designed to allow emergency suppression of therapy, but the modes vary between manufacturers. Magnet mode in Guidant devices can be programmed either on—the device will allow temporary suspension of therapy or inactivation of the ICD, or off—a magnet has no effect. The magnet mode of ICDs from Medtronic and Ventritex always suspends detection and tachycardia therapy. Antibradycardia pacing is not affected.

MYOCARDIAL INFARCTION (MI)

Another complex term that simply means "a heart attack". After prolonged ischemia (lack of oxygen) the tissue dies and is then called an infarct. The myocardial tissue is the heart muscle. So myocardial infarction describes dead heart muscle, which often results in death, but can also cause arrhythmias from the scar tissue.

NON-INVASIVE PROGRAMMED STIMULATION (NIPS)

A term used in hospitals for "testing the ICD". The goal of this testing is to evaluate the ICD system and assess its program for treatment of dangerous arrhythmias. It is non invasive, in that the body is not pierced to perform the test, but it is personally invasive in that ventricular fibrillation is deliberately induced in the patient under clinical conditions, and requires defibrillation to restore a normal rhythm.

PREMATURE VENTRICULAR CONTRACTION (PVC)

Preventricular Contractions, Premature Ventricular Complexes or Premature Ventricular Contractions are sometimes felt as "skipped beats". They are extra electrical impulses arising from one of the cardiac ventricles, unlike a normal heartbeat that starts in the atria.

You may have felt your heart "skip a beat" for no reason. The heart doesn't really skip a beat; rather a beat (contraction) comes sooner than normal (premature). Then there is a pause that causes the next beat to be more forceful, which feels like a thump after a pause; hence the term "skipping a beat". These premature beats are most often the cause of irregular heart rhythms, and are often called palpitations. Few cardiac arrhythmias have created as much consternation and confusion, among both doctors and patients, as PVCs.

Palpitations are a common complaint that many people describe as a skipping, pounding, fluttering, flip-flopping, racing, or sudden stopping of the heartbeat. You may feel your heart speed up when you climb a flight of stairs or drink too much coffee. The rapid beating may last for seconds, minutes or even hours. While many people with palpitations can ignore them, others find them extremely disturbing and frightening, and often worry that they are about to die at any moment.

PVCs are the most common arrhythmia found in a cardiac catheterization laboratory. They are the result of ectopic foci (abnormal point of origin), electrically stimulating the entire ventricular wall to contract out of synchronization with the electrical stimulation of the SA node. The PVC appears as a wide, aberrant QRS complex. There is no P-wave because the electrical impulse for contraction did not originate from the SA node.

There are specific names given to represent the number of PVCs presented on an electrocardiogram. Bigeminy is the name given to PVCs that occur after every QRS complex (i.e., every other beat is a PVC). Trigeminy defines those PVCs that occur after every second beat (i.e., two QRS complexes followed by a PVC). The term Quadgeminy describes a PVC every fourth beat. PVCs can also be characterized by the similarity in the shape of the QRS complex. Unifocal PVCs are those that originate from the same ectopic foci in the ventricle. The shape of each PVC wave is similar. Multifocal PVCs originate from two or more ectopic foci in the ventricle. These ectopic foci can be located anywhere in the ventricles, and can occur sporadically, displaying a unique shape in all the electrocardiogram leads. PVCs are considered dangerous and life threatening if there are more than five occurring in a one minute period or if they are multifocal.

Since PVCs can occur at anytime during the electrical conduction of the heart, the action potential of myocardial contraction can also be affected. In other words, PVCs can trigger an irregular heart rhythm. PVCs that occur during the normal T-wave are called an "R on T" events. Since the T-wave represents ventricular repolarization, it is during this stage of the action potential of the ventricle that the muscle is susceptible to any external stimulation that would cause contraction. Ectopic foci can create a stimulus that can overwhelm the ventricular musculature and result in an arrhythmia. An "R on T" event can cause a resulting arrhythmia that may progress into V-tach, or even V-fib. Carolyn's electrophysiologist suggested this is what may have occurred in October 2002. But no one will ever know for sure!

ACKNOWLEDGEMENTS

*Many of life's greatest failures are people who
did not realize how close they were to success when they gave up.*
                                                        –Thomas A. Edison

Without the care and dedication of the following people, Carolyn would not be alive and well. We are grateful and appreciative of their professionalism and humanity, especially to those who do not deal with the issues of sudden cardiac arrest in their normal daily life.

I want to mention and acknowledge the efforts of those special people in the room with Carolyn that day; those who maintained her "furnace of life" until medical help arrived. Without them, she would have been just another statistic.

THE SAVIORS
   Tom O'Brien
   Randy Fitch
   Kathy Williams –Director of Education, Denton Regional Hospital

And in recognition of those whose care and attention to detail ensured Carolyn was looked after as a family member.

THE BOSS
   Jim Hardee
THE COLLEAGUES
   Pam Battistone
   Karen Davey
   Bruce Senecal

The EMTs are under the greatest pressure to perform in less than ideal conditions, and with little or no time to consider alternative therapies. They are remarkable for their reliability and diligence. Carolyn was more than lucky to have this crew attend to her, and we are grateful that they achieved their second "save".

GRAPEVINE RESCUE, STATION 5 CREW
Tom Humes
Jeff Jackson
Chris Lammons
Carl Nix
Stephen Sheffield

The doctors may feel they were just doing their job, but it means a lot to me that they had the skills and the determination to help Carolyn survive and recover.

BAYLOR GRAPEVINE HOSPITAL
Dr. David Diamond –ER
Dr. Martin Soloman –Neurology
Dr. Jackie Preston –Internist
Dr. Phillip Hecht –Cardiology
Dr. James Siminski –Pulmonology

BAYLOR HEART & VASCULAR HOSPITAL
Dr. Peter John Wells –Electrophysiology
Dr. Kevin Robert Wheelan –Cardiology

The people who need a special mention are the ones we have limited records of. They are the real caregivers—the nurses. While we don't have all their details, we remember their attention, dedication and care. They are such special people, and their actions will not be forgotten.

ASSOCIATIONS

As a general rule the most successful man in life
is the man who has the best information.

—Disraeli

American Heart Association (AHA)
Reducing disability and death from cardiovascular diseases and stroke, and the Go Red For Women heart disease awareness movement. CPR Line Phone: (888) 277-5463   http://www.americanheart.org

Sudden Cardiac Arrest Foundation (SCAF)
Raising Awareness, saving lives. The Sudden Cardiac Arrest Foundation is an independent, non-profit center of excellence focused on reducing death and disability from sudden cardiac arrest.

http://www.sca-aware.org

American Red Cross (ARC)
Red Cross Preparedness programs in first aid, CPR and AED are available for any age and can be tailored to the needs of specific groups and individuals.   http://www.redcross.org

Heart Rhythm Society (HRS)
The Heart Rhythm Society represents the specialties of cardiac pacing and cardiac electrophysiology. It is active on issues of cardiac arrhythmia management, such as Medicare reimbursement, federal oversight on the safety and effectiveness of medical devices, and guidelines for medical practice in the pacemaker, electrophysiologic, and patient communities.

http://www.hrsonline.org

BIBLIOGRAPHY & ATTRIBUTIONS

*Let the young know they will never find a more interesting,
more instructive book than the patient himself.*

–Giorgio Baglivi

Mickey S. Eisenberg, *Life in the balance:* New York, Oxford University Press, 1997.

Deborah Daw Heffernan, *An Arrow through the Heart:* Free Press Simon & Schuster, 2002.

Robert McCrum, *My Year Off:* W. W. Norton & Company, 1998.

Wayne M. Sotile, *Thriving with Heart Disease:* Free Press Simon & Schuster, 2003.

Larry Dossey, *Healing Words:* HarperCollins, 1993.

Trisha Meili, *I am the New York Jogger:* Scribner, 2003.

Susan L. Woods, *Cardiac Nursing:* Lippincott Williams & Wilkins, 2000.

About the Author

In 2002, Jeremy Whitehead came to America, fulfilling a life-long dream. That dream changed, however, when his wife suffered a cardiac arrest within six weeks of their wedding day. After researching the causes and consequences of Sudden Cardiac Arrest, Jeremy realized that many others want to understand what it is, why it happens and what to do about it. He interviewed the saviors and witnesses to Carolyn's collapse—to capture their thoughts and feelings at the time—and found they, too, were profoundly affected by the event. It is for those yet to be touched by this well understood but incurable leading cause of death, that he decided to share their story.

http://www.heart2good.com

Jeremy has been a public advocate volunteer for the American Heart Association and the Sudden Cardiac Arrest Foundation. In 2004, he was instrumental in convincing Congress to approve further funding of defibrillators. He has been published in the *Journal of Emergency Medical Services* (JEMS March, 2005).

Jeremy graduated as an electronics engineer in the telecommunications industry, and excelled at marketing the Internet. He then moved to IBM Software Group. He has a reputation for mastering complex subjects, and making them simple to understand.

Now a freelance writer, and a graduate of the Australian College of Journalism, Jeremy is focused on narrative nonfiction and the self-help genre. Born in Australia, Jeremy now lives with his wife in Westchester County, New York.   http://www.jeremywhitehead.com